Sally-Ann Creed is the author of nine books, including the bestselling *Let Food Be Your Medicine*, which is still viewed as a classic today.

Having spent her early years in and out of ICU units, suffering from chronic illness, and her 20s battling an ever-escalating list of ailments, Creed found herself on dozens of medications, seeing innumerable doctors and specialists, and undergoing endless tests and thirteen sinus operations.

After decades of searching for a stable sense of medical wellbeing, it wasn't until Dr Robbie Simons gave Creed back her health and her life that she decided to study the subject further. She went on to achieve a postgraduate diploma in Clinical Nutrition and later studied Functional Medicine.

OTHER BOOKS BY
SALLY-ANN CREED INCLUDE:

- *Let Food Be Your Medicine*, bestseller 2002, 2004, 2006.

- *Nutritious*, co-authored with the late
Jill Fraser Halkett.

- *Woman's Health Journal*, co-authored
with Aldyth Thomson.

- *Raising Healthy Happy Children*, co-authored with
Andalene Salvesen.

- *The Real Meal Revolution*, co-authored with Tim Noakes,
David Grier and Jonno Proudfoot – winner of the Nielsen
Booksellers Choice Award, Book of the Year 2014.
International version of the above – now globally released
in several languages.

- *Die Kos Revolusie*, with above authors, 2014.

- *Tasty WasteNots*, co-authored with Jason Whitehead,
released in 2016 , winner of the national Gourmand
World Cookbook Award in the Innovative category, 2017.

- *Delicious Low Carb*, 2016.

- *Lekker Low Carb*, 2016.

THE LOW-CARB, HEALTHY FAT BIBLE

SALLY-ANN CREED

Co-author of the bestselling *The Real Meal Revolution*

ROBINSON

ROBINSON

First published in South Africa in 2016 by Creed Nutrition

First published in Great Britain in 2018 by Robinson

1 3 5 7 9 10 8 6 4 2

A CIP catalogue record for this book
is available from the British Library.

ISBN: 978-1-47214-098-2

Printed and Bound in Great Britain by Bell and Bain Ltd, Glasgow

Papers used by Robinson are from well-managed forests
and other responsible sources.

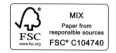

Robinson
An imprint of
Little, Brown Book Group
Carmelite House
50 Victoria Embankment
London EC4Y 0DZ

An Hachette UK Company
www.hachette.co.uk

www.littlebrown.co.uk

THE
LOW-CARB,
HEALTHY FAT
BIBLE

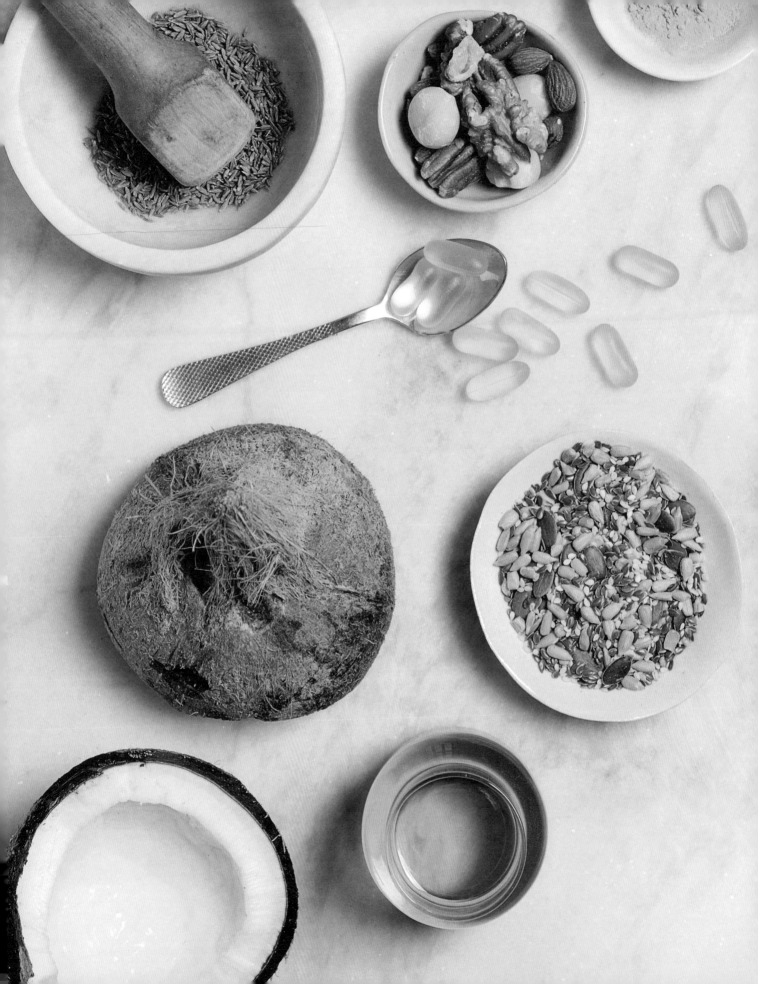

CONTENTS

INTRODUCTION

Out of intense complexities intense simplicities emerge.

– Winston Churchill

HOW IT ALL BEGAN

I first met Tim in early March 2013. After our meeting, he tweeted, calling me "South Africa's first Paleo nutritionist". This got the attention of a young chef who approached me to write a cookbook along the lines of the LCHF lifestyle. I nearly refused, but eventually agreed to write the lifestyle and diet aspect of the book to complement the recipes. I suggested that we should invite Tim to join us and David came on board as the second chef.

We decided that the lifestyle should be called Banting. It was named after the illustrious English undertaker, William Banting, who published his *Letter on Corpulence* in the mid-1800s, which documented his extensive weight loss achieved through lifestyle change. Dieters who followed his guidance were called Banters.

Our book, *The Real Meal Revolution* (referred to hereafter as 'the red book'), came out in South Africa within a few months. It became a bestseller, winning the 2014 Nielsen Booksellers' Choice Award for Book of the Year, and is now published internationally. I coined the term "changing the way a nation eats" shortly thereafter. The nation grabbed the idea with both hands: hundreds of thousands of people lost weight, and it literally changed the way South Africa ate. A revolution began.

Within a short time, entrepreneurs climbed aboard the phenomenon and launched new businesses:

restaurants and cottage industries mushroomed, social media pages burgeoned overnight, and soon Banting products of every description hit the shelves. However, many merely traded on the word "Banting", creating products that had little to do with the lifestyle. There was money to be made, and the honest and unscrupulous together began to rake it in. This is one of the reasons we'll refer to this lifestyle from here on as low-carbohydrate healthy fat (LCHF).

From a personal standpoint, the whole thrust of the red book came from a simple desire to teach people to eat real food cooked from scratch, rather than processed food. This has been my passion for 23 years. Balance was called for – not excess. During this time, as the book's nutritional author, I became so inundated with enquiries that I decided to put together a six-month course which contained all the knowledge I had gleaned from 20 years of clinical practice and research.

The demand for support was so unrelenting that I created a nationwide network of coaches, chosen from those who had taken my course, to spread the burden. After students completed the course and two days of intensive hands-on training with myself and an administrative training partner, they did a sterling job of counselling people in the paradigm. My partner subsequently took over the business, and the two contributing authors of this book – Merle and Janita – are from the first intake of trainee coaches.

In response to the term "Banting" losing its meaning, it has become necessary to clarify what it *really* was meant to be and what it is *not*. I also want to briefly introduce the Paleo lifestyle, which may suit some people better than the stricter LCHF – the choice is yours. In the following pages, I will demonstrate the advantages of LCHF as it was envisaged originally, with certain modifications as required in light of ongoing research, and hopefully answer questions along the way. It's impossible to cram everything into one book, but I've tried my best.

LCHF is the perfect lifestyle for hunger-free weight loss. It corrects metabolic syndrome and brings the body back to its set point and ideal mass. You can follow this programme and stick to it if it continues to work for you, or gradually move into the Paleo lifestyle, with its subtle changes. I wish to make plain that the core message is, and always will be, eat real food: food as close to nature as possible, and in accordance with **The Creed**.

Please note: Nothing in this book is in any way prescriptive (please see the disclaimer on page 244). I do not pretend to be an expert as I do not believe such a creature exists. I acknowledge that nobody has all the truth. I hope this book will complement the red book and fill in some gaps.

Welcome to the low-carb revolution – it's a fabulous lifestyle.

MISSION STATEMENT

In this book, I endeavour to clear up confusion, answer some pressing questions and present new ideas. I hope that both seasoned LCHF enthusiasts and new converts to the lifestyle will benefit from the information in this book. Please note that while I concentrate primarily on the Banting angle (defined as the lifestyle as laid out in the red book and now called LCHF), this book also seeks to cover the wider low-carb paradigm.

To clarify what is meant by a LCHF lifestyle:

- It is primarily about eating *real* food, not processed food or junk food.
- It avoids low-carb treats to focus on nutritious whole food; treats are very occasional.
- A healthy lifestyle by default includes fresh, natural food, which means leaving out *all* commercial sauces, foods and the usual boxed and bottled things you buy. Focused LCHF enthusiasts who truly understand the meaning of this lifestyle will make their own food from scratch.
- Saturated fat is healthy and has been wrongfully vilified. It is in fact a healthy superfood.
- Foods should be full fat, never 'lite', low-fat or fat-free. Often reduced fat products contain sugar, some sort of sweetener or other additives to give palatability. Important fats in the diet include all the animal fats available including grass-fed butter – fat is not the enemy here.
- Margarine and all seed oils are processed, man-made substitutes for healthy fat. They are inflammatory, unstable and harmful to the human body – I do *not* recommend any of them at all at any time in any shape or form. LCHF shuns *all* seed and grain oils of any description, and margarines.
- Cholesterol is a healthy and much-needed substance made by the human body for a vast array of bodily functions. It is not disease-causing – without cholesterol we would die.
- Refined carbohydrates are not only inflammatory, addictive and cause weight gain, but they now appear to be linked to a number of dread diseases such as cardiovascular disease, diabetes and even cancers.
- All forms of sugar and artificial sweeteners should be avoided.
- Fructose is unhealthy and harmful. It is metabolised by the body in a way that can lead to fatty liver, diabetes, gout, cardiovascular disease and obesity.
- Agave is almost pure fructose, and should be avoided completely.
- Exercise is encouraged and recommended, but studies indicate it does nothing to cause weight loss. However, it is helpful for improving insulin sensitivity and we recommend exercise if you are able to do it; particularly high-intensity interval training.
- Microwaved food, convenience food, take-away food and anything processed is frowned

upon as unnatural and abnormal –
healthy LCHF followers wouldn't
dream of consuming any of these.

- Genetically modified organisms
  (GMO) are totally outlawed in this
  lifestyle. My recommendations are always
  pasture-fed, organic or at least free
  range, and meats which don't contain
  hormones, steroids, antibiotics
  or growth promoters.
- Various foods like soya, maize and
  legumes are not consumed in
  this paradigm.
- I regard plastic as harmful, especially
  when it comes into contact with any kind
  of fat or oil medium, and especially a soft
  plastic that can be squeezed.

....

*Please note: I do not recommend
you change your diet without your
doctor's supervision, or if you are
pregnant, breastfeeding, an infant,
a young child or are infirm – or
indeed if you have any questions
about this lifestyle whatsoever.
I recommend that anyone with any
health condition contacts a qualified
health professional for medical
advice.*

THE CREED

1. **Eat healthy fat.** Choose from the healthy fats
   list. Eat only fats found in nature, never the
   man-made processed versions.
2. **Avoid seed and grain oils.** All seed and grain
   oils are off limits to a serious low-carb, real
   food adherent. We believe no seed or grain
   oils are healthy.
3. **No sugar in any form.** This includes agave,
   fructose and all other forms of sugar.
4. **No grains.** Your love affair with grains has
   lasted too long – it's time to cut the cord!
   Grains can seriously harm your digestive tract,
   raise blood sugar and prevent weight loss.
5. **Eat *quality* protein.** Aim for pasture-fed
   animal protein if possible, always humanely
   reared; including eggs, poultry and wild-caught
   fish. No antibiotics or growth promoters
   should be used.
6. **Eat enough protein.** But not too much.
   A portion is the size and shape of the
   palm and thickness of your hand. This is
   a moderate, not a high protein lifestyle.
7. **Avoid harmful foods.** Avoid soya, legumes
   and processed food. Also avoid all chemicals
   in foods – they are unnatural and
   extremely harmful.
8. **No fizzy, soft or fruit drinks.** Liquid sugar and
   artificial sweeteners are all no-nos.
9. **Avoid fruit.** Avoid or limit – it's another form
   of sugar.
10. **Eat your vegetables.** These are vital for
    fibre content, valuable antioxidants
    and phytonutrients.
11. **No snacking.** In the first week you may if you
    think you might die, but you won't. Protein and

fat will keep you satisfied for longer, so there is no need to keep blood sugar and insulin constantly elevated. Instead of snacking, eat two to three proper meals a day.

12. **Don't binge.** You cannot throw caution to the wind and eat all you like on a low-carb lifestyle. Control food intake without obsession, so stop eating when you are 80 per cent full.

13. **Don't starve.** Under-eating will slow your metabolism. This is about balance, sustainability, and eating in a healthy, sensible way – it's not supposed to be torture.

14. **Eat to hunger, not routine.** Mealtimes with family are fine, but mindless grazing all day long isn't – you aren't a cow. Eat two to three good meals a day, and don't snack in between.

15. **Don't be misled.** Avoid commercial LCHF products for the most part, they are usually not low-carb by any stretch of the imagination. Just make your own and avoid the processed stuff, or at the very least read labels and ask leading questions.

16. **Be discriminating about dairy.** Many people have problems with dairy. Read the reasons why dairy may be problematic for you personally in this lifestyle.

17. **Limit nuts.** Technically, nuts are allowed in this lifestyle; but go easy – they're high in inflammatory omega-6 oils so eating too many will prevent weight loss. Limit your intake, and activate them first if possible.

18. **Avoid alcohol.** You have to 'live a little' and I don't want to spoil your fun! However, a healthy lifestyle doesn't include daily alcohol, nor excess. It may prevent weight loss for up to three days after a drink (especially in women). The choice is yours.

19. **No microwaves please!** Cook on a stove or in an oven, never in a microwave, which denatures food and destroys vital nutrients.

20. **It's all about *real* food.** *Never* forget that. NO processed food, takeaways or fake versions of the real thing. In a nutshell: no junk. I support single-ingredient foods, put together at home with love and passion.

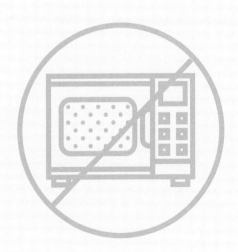

01

LAYING THE FOUNDATION

*The diet-heart hypothesis that suggests that high intake of saturated fat and cholesterol causes heart disease has been repeatedly shown to be wrong, and yet, for complicated reasons of pride, profit and prejudice, the hypothesis continues to be exploited by scientists, fund-raising enterprises, food companies, and even government agencies. The public is being deceived by the **greatest health scam of the century**.*

– Dr George Mann, ScD, MD, Former Co-Director, The Framingham Study

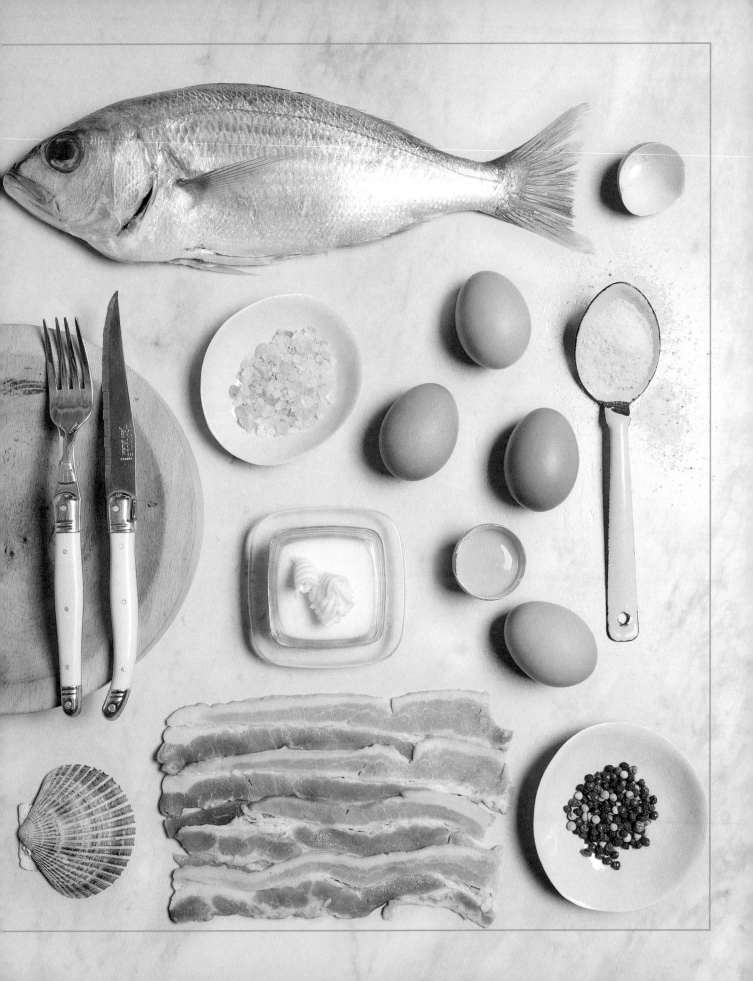

Chapter

01

THE HORMONE CONNECTION

In order to fully understand how a successful low-carb lifestyle works, it's important to understand the dietary science behind this way of eating.

INSULIN.

When it comes to weight loss, you really only have to know about insulin and how to keep it low. If you understand the role of insulin in the body and respond accordingly, you will solve your weight management problems. In a nutshell: the lower your insulin levels, the more successful your weight loss.

Insulin is a hormone, or chemical messenger, which is released from the pancreas into the bloodstream in response to a meal. Insulin ensures that all of the sugars, amino acids and fatty acids that are released from digested and absorbed meals are taken up by cells of the body. Insulin acts like a doorman: it attaches to the cells and causes little channels to open to let glucose in. It also allows certain amino acids to enter muscle cells and fatty acids to enter the adipocytes (fat cells).

The immediate function of glucose in all cells is energy supply. If there is any glucose left after energy needs are met, the liver converts the excess glucose to glycogen. Once the glycogen reserves are full, the remaining glucose is converted to fat. These fats are transported to the adipocytes and stored there.

Insulin is responsible for this deposition of fat and more importantly, for locking it away. The fat will be released from the adipocytes only if the insulin levels are very low. So if you want to empty your fat cells in the pursuit of weight loss, your eating behaviour must be such as to keep insulin levels very low at all times.

This is the secret of low-carb living – it translates into low blood insulin levels.

GLUCAGON.

Another hormone secreted from the pancreas should be mentioned briefly because it has the opposite effect on glucose to that of insulin. If the blood sugar level drops below about 80 milligrams per 100 millilitres, glucagon is released to convert the stored glucose (glycogen) in the liver back into free glucose, ensuring that there is always enough glucose in the blood for the body's energy needs. If the blood sugar level is not maintained in this way, one of the first signs of such hypoglycaemia would be loss of consciousness, since the brain is the most voracious user of blood glucose. This is if you are not keto-adapted, in which case the brain needs less glucose.

High-carb eating, particularly snacking, wreaks havoc on blood sugar levels; straight after a meal, blood glucose levels shoot up, and insulin rushes in to bring it down to normal, safe levels. However, when too much insulin is released, too much glucose is removed from the blood, resulting in a state of hypoglycaemia. Glucagon should be released in response to this hypoglycaemia, but so much insulin is produced in response to the dietary sugar onslaught that the glucagon cannot override it and the low blood sugar state stimulates the hunger centre in the brain, leading to the desire to eat again. Usually, the food eaten in response to this hunger is high in carbohydrates (carbs), and so the insulin just remains high all day, and the cycle is repeated with every snack.

Remember the golden rule: as long as insulin is around, fat will not be released from the fat cells. You have to find out how many grams of carbs your body can take per day so that your insulin levels are low enough to allow fat to be set free. This is the secret of low-carb dieting – keeping the carbs low means keeping the insulin low. The low-carb lifestyle means that fat can be released easily from storage as an alternative to glucose for your daily fuel needs.

INSULIN RESISTANCE AND DIABETES.

If the pancreas is unable to make insulin, it is usually the first sign of Type 1 diabetes. The cause is not fully understood: genetics, stress, the environment, viruses and auto-immunity are all blamed for causing Type 1 diabetes. Sufferers of Type 1 diabetes have to take insulin injections for the rest of their lives.

Type 2 diabetes, on the other hand, is caused by insulin resistance – it is a 'lifestyle disease' characterised by both high blood glucose and insulin levels. Normally, high insulin should bring about low glucose readings, so clearly the insulin is not working if both levels are high. What seems to be happening is the pancreas, being constantly aware of a high blood sugar level, pumps out more insulin. The blood sugar does not come down, so the pancreas sends more insulin, and so on.

Glucose builds up in the blood, which becomes too sugary or hyperglycaemic – this is the first sign of diabetes, whether it be Type 1 or Type 2. The ravages of diabetes on the body are due to excessive amounts of glucose in the blood, which has a damaging effect on small blood vessels so that the kidneys are damaged, vision is impaired and there is loss of sensation in the extremities (neuropathy), among other problems.

What causes the muscle, and particularly the liver cells of the body, to resist the effect of insulin? Researchers have found that the cells begin to lose their insulin receptors. These are special sites on the cells' surfaces which allow insulin to attach and do its work of opening the channels to admit glucose. They gradually decrease in number, so no matter how much insulin there is, the receptors cannot do their work and so the sugar just builds up, unusable.

Why does this happen? It has been suggested that the excessive amount of glucose entering the cells associated with a high-carb diet is actually toxic, and so the cells begin to shun the overload by removing their insulin receptors.

The adipocytes of the abdomen, in the growing environment of high glucose and insulin within the body, become over-stimulated, making and storing fat in excess, meaning obesity is associated with insulin resistance. Along with abdominal obesity, other metabolic disturbances associated with heart disease are manifested: blood pressure goes up, triglycerides (fat) in the bloodstream rises, HDL (the so-called good cholesterol) goes down and a dangerous species of small, dense particle LDL goes up. If the constantly raised blood sugar levels prevail, diabetes can result. These combined problems are referred to as metabolic syndrome.

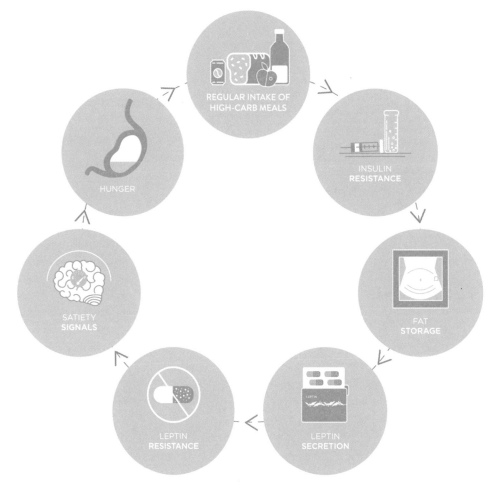

Inspired by www.primalprotein.com

HYPERINSULINAEMIA.

Hyperinsulinaemia (high blood insulin) causes blood pressure and triglycerides to increase, as well as creating other problems. Fat tissue now becomes an inflammatory 'organ' as the expanding cells release chemicals called cytokines, causing inflammation throughout the body. Apart from damaging the kidneys' ability to control blood pressure, the excretion of uric acid is also impaired, and this can lead to gout.

Arteries become less elastic with all this insulin, and together with the inflammatory cytokines and the toxic effect of hyperglycaemia, this can lead to damage to their inner lining. The small LDL particles, which arise as a result of metabolic syndrome, are attracted to the damaged artery wall lining, where they act as a sort of plaster to protect the tear in the artery lining. In the process, they form the beginnings of atheromas (fatty plaques), which develop into full-blown artery disease, or arteriosclerosis. There is also now evidence to suggest that Alzheimer's disease is a result of years of dysregulated glucose; the term Type 3 diabetes is applied to the dementia caused by sugar. Poorly controlled diabetics would automatically be much more prone to this form of dementia.

GHRELIN AND LEPTIN.

These hormones regulate satiety. Ghrelin is released from the stomach and is associated with hunger, while leptin is released from the fat cells in response to a meal. Both hormones affect the same part of the brain, with ghrelin signalling the need for food and leptin giving the 'stop eating' signal.

If soft drinks containing fructose are consumed with food, the fructose tends to block the action of leptin; and more food can be eaten because there is no feeling of satiety. It has been found that high levels of insulin in the blood, as occur in insulin resistance, *block* the action of leptin so insulin resistance is accompanied by hunger as the brain cannot 'see' the leptin. Insulin resistance is therefore accompanied by leptin resistance. There are no products which can mimic leptin or suppress ghrelin to help people lose weight, don't be fooled.

CORTISOL.

Cortisol is a stress hormone. Its job is to sustain you through short episodes of stress such as a car accident. If your adrenal glands are unable to produce cortisol during an accident, this alone could kill you, quite apart from the effects of any injuries you may suffer.

The function of cortisol during stressful emergencies is to raise blood sugar and fats as well as blood pressure. These should return to normal quickly after the event. If, however, stress becomes prolonged and unmanageable (certain people cannot deal with prolonged stress), then cortisol levels remain high.

Over time, stress has the effect of reducing leptin sensitivity and raising ghrelin so that you develop a desire particularly for comfort foods, which are usually high-carb, highly calorific fatty foods and sweet things. Stressed people also often experience reduced sleep time, which is associated with systemic inflammation. Because of the reduced leptin and increased ghrelin, the cortisol becomes a contributing factor in the development of metabolic syndrome.

Excessive cortisol exposure working alongside hyperinsulinaemia results characteristically in the deposition of abdominal fat.

KETOSIS.

This is the condition the body is in when the bulk of its energy requirements are supplied by fuel molecules called ketones and free fatty acids (FFA). These fuels are derived from the breakdown of the fat stored in the body and dietary fat when you switch from a carbohydrate-rich diet to LCHF eating. That is why ketosis, and therefore the LCHF lifestyle, is associated with weight loss.

Opponents or critics of the LCHF approach and the associated ketosis of healthy people in a fat-burning mode confuse ketosis with the life-threatening ketoacidosis of uncontrolled diabetics and alcoholics. The blood is normally kept at a very precise, slightly alkaline pH of 7.4 by its own buffering ability and by the kidneys and lungs. In diabetic and alcoholic ketoacidosis, the ketone output is about 400 times that of a fully keto-adapted healthy person, and this tips the blood towards a pH of 7.2 and below, which can be fatal if sustained for a long period of time. The ketosis experienced on a LCHF regimen produces about 115 grams to 180 grams of ketones per day, whereas diabetic ketoacidosis generates over 400 grams per day.

The LCHF level of ketosis is associated with excellent physical and mental well-being. Healthy people have a safety mechanism to stop ketosis from getting out of control, unlike diabetics. At a certain point, if ketones become too elevated in the blood, insulin secretion is stimulated, which stops the liver from making more ketones and reconstructs the ketones back into fat molecules, to be stored away in the fat cells – out of harm's way.

Type 1 diabetics cannot produce insulin so this does not happen for them. The kidneys also excrete excess ketones. The scaremongering about ketosis is therefore groundless.

Ketosis was actually used to treat childhood epilepsy until drugs came along. Those children experienced no ill-effects from ketosis, so why should adults seeking to lose weight suddenly be at risk?

Please note: Having said this, I do not routinely recommend that you go into ketosis, as you are well able to sustain weight loss at much higher levels of carbohydrate intake. This is merely for those who wish to do so or who require understanding of the term. Eating 50 grams of carbs a day or less can induce ketosis. However, most people will need to drop to around 25 grams of carbs per day.

How ketosis works.

On day one of ketosis, all your glycogen (stored glucose in the liver and muscles) is used up, and within three days on a LCHF diet, your insulin levels will be sustained low enough (owing to your low-carb status) to allow fat to be released from the fat cells. The liver will first break up each fat molecule into three FFAs and one glycerol molecule. It will then chop some of the large fatty acids into tiny ketone bodies for easy combustion in the cells. Glycerol is turned into glucose which is used to fuel those tissues (blood cells and bone marrow) which cannot use ketones or FFA for fuel. You will have switched from being largely glucose-fuelled to being fat-fuelled. Using a car analogy, this is like changing from relatively dirty diesel power to pure, clean, efficient hydrogen power.

Tissues such as bone marrow and blood cells use glucose only for fuel and the body will always make enough glucose for these from the glycerol, which is released when fat is broken down, and some of the proteins in the diet (or your own muscle if you are actually starving). All other tissues function very well on ketones and even plain FFA, which are pushed out by the liver from both adipocyte and dietary sources.

It is important to eat protein when on a LCHF diet, otherwise the body will break down its own protein to make glucose and you will suffer muscle loss. About 15 grams of protein a day is enough to prevent this from happening.

It is a misconception that the brain can only operate on glucose. It takes about three weeks for the brain to switch over to ketone power and it has a 25 per cent need for glucose thereafter, which is adequately supplied from the conversion of amino acids from dietary protein and glycerol to glucose in the liver. It is interesting to note that during the three weeks the brain is changing over to ketones, the other tissues of the body, especially the muscles, use ketones: but when the brain is fully keto-adapted, it ends up hogging most of the ketones and the rest of the body uses FFA for fuel. During ketosis, the triglyceride level in the blood tends to drop from its pre-ketosis state as triglycerides are being used by the liver to make ketones and FFA and glucose.

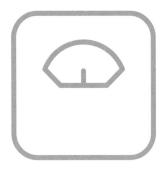

The best way to measure the effects of a LCHF lifestyle on your body is not necessarily with Ketostix strips, which search for ketones in the urine, or breath analysis, which looks for acetone, as these are all notoriously unreliable indicators of what is really going on in the body. The best way to measure your progress is with the bathroom scales, the tape measure and skin-fold measurements. A static weight may mean you are replacing fat with muscle and the absence of acetone on the breath does not mean you are not in ketosis.

Best of all is to see how your body changes in your clothing. Is it looser and feeling too big for you? All is then on track; who cares what the scales say.

GLUCONEOGENESIS.

At all times the body needs to maintain a certain blood glucose level of about 80 milligrams of glucose per 100 millilitres of blood, because the brain and other tissues like red blood cells always need some glucose. Even when one is fully keto-adapted this remains true. So how does the body maintain a blood glucose level on a zero-carb diet? The answer is gluconeogenesis (literally: the 'generation of new glucose'). The liver and kidneys are able to convert certain amino acids into glucose. There are always amino acids circulating in the blood and these organs simply grab some of these when blood glucose is low, and chemically convert them into glucose – it is as simple as that.

Another starter molecule for gluconeogenesis in the liver is glycerol. When in ketosis, the fats released from fat cells are broken down into one glycerol molecule and three fatty acids. The fatty acids are used instead of glucose in a keto-adapted person and the glycerol is converted into glucose to help maintain the blood glucose level.

Gluconeogenesis is controlled by the pancreas, which releases the hormone glucagon when blood sugars are low, and this glucagon tells the liver and kidneys to start the process of gluconeogenesis. Glucagon is also responsible for glycogenolysis, which is the release of stored glucose from glycogen, but this happens only when one is on a high-carb diet where excess glucose from the food eaten gets stored as glycogen. This happens between meals to maintain blood sugar levels.

CHOLESTEROL.

Cholesterol means different things to different people, and there is much confusion as a result. Firstly, the actual chemical substance called cholesterol is a single molecule that is made in the liver and is so important that you cannot live without it for many reasons.

It is found in cell membranes surrounding every single cell in the body, forming many of the tiny machines called organelles within the cells. Cholesterol is also the precursor to many important steroid hormones in the body like progesterone, testosterone, aldosterone, cortisol and the oestrogens. Sunlight converts cholesterol in the skin fat to the hormone cholecalciferol (also known as Vitamin D3).

Cholesterol is excreted from the body by the liver in the form of bile salts, which are released from the gall bladder after meals and attach to digested fat from the intestine in order to transport the fat into the blood. They are responsible for the absorption of fat. In other words, you reabsorb the bile salts and this means that up to 50 per cent of your cholesterol is recycled.

If cholesterol were such a dangerous substance worthy of being blocked by statins, why then does your liver produce it and why do you reabsorb it from the gut to be recycled?

The name 'cholesterol' is also applied to a large variety of particles found in the blood. These particles contain millions upon millions of molecules of cholesterol, some fats called phospholipids and still other fats called triglycerides. Triglycerides and cholesterol are insoluble in the watery plasma of the blood (fat floats on water), so in order to dissolve in the plasma and be carried around the body, these particles are surrounded by water-soluble

phospholipids, proteins and antioxidant molecules (protecting the fats from going rancid).

The whole spherical particle that is formed is called a lipoprotein. These lipoproteins are unfortunately also called 'cholesterol' which can be a little confusing. To add to the confusion, there are many different kinds of lipoproteins (or cholesterol): there are the high-density lipoproteins (HDL) and the low-density lipoproteins (LDL) and just for the record, there are VLDLs and IDLs too (very low density and intermediate density). To add to the confusion, there are different kinds of proteins and different sizes of these various particles: the most important particles to consider are the big and the small LDL cholesterols.

Put simply, this is what happens: the liver makes and then puts large 'fluffy' LDLs into the blood to be carried all over the body, where the cholesterols and triglycerides and phospholipids are offloaded to be used by the tissues. The LDLs get smaller and denser, resulting in one of two kinds – large (pattern A) types and small (pattern B) types. The small pattern B LDLs have more triglycerides on board than the pattern A LDLs, and they arise as a result of insulin resistance and a high-carbohydrate diet containing sugar and processed foods.

It so happens that if the artery wall is damaged and little injuries in the lining of the artery occur due to inflammation (from sugar and high insulin levels), the pattern B LDLs are small enough to slip into these tiny tears in the wall and accumulate almost as if to protect the damaged area. The larger pattern A LDLs are too big to join in and they do

TWO PATIENTS WITH THE SAME LDL-C
WHO IS AT RISK?

———

At the <u>**same level of LDL cholesterol**</u>, people with small LDLs can
have **up to 70%** more particles than people with large LDLs.

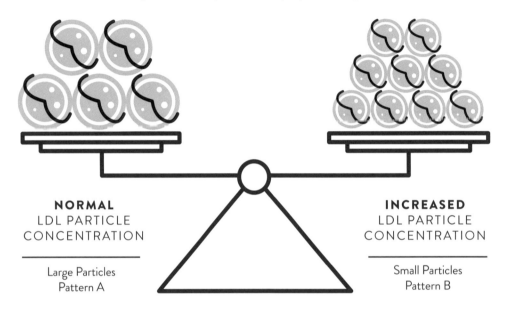

NORMAL
LDL PARTICLE
CONCENTRATION

———

Large Particles
Pattern A

INCREASED
LDL PARTICLE
CONCENTRATION

———

Small Particles
Pattern B

Inspired by Dr Daniel Dayspring

not contribute to the ensuing disease process: in time, fatty streaks begin to grow as more small LDLs, particularly those with oxidised cholesterol accumulate in the plaque. They become engulfed by white blood cells within the artery wall, forming foam cells and eventually porridge-like atheromas develop.

Muscle cells begin to grow from the artery wall into this area and calcium is deposited to make the whole thing a hardened mass or plaque, blocking the artery. As long as this plaque is stable, there is only the inconvenience of a

compromised blood flow to the organ concerned; but if the plaque surface ruptures, the exposed gunk attracts blood platelets which form a clot. Now the artery is totally blocked, causing a heart attack or stroke.

LCHF and exercise should very successfully prevent the formation of small, dense pattern B LDLs because sugar and processed foods are avoided and insulin resistance is reversed. Avoiding sugar also prevents the cholesterols from being glycated (sugar-coated), which makes them suitable only for making plaque.

You should similarly protect all your lipoproteins by maintaining good dietary antioxidant status and supplementing with Vitamins C and E, coenzyme Q10 and plenty of flavonoids (from red and blue pigmented vegetables and berries). Pattern B LDLs oxidise and glycate more readily than pattern A LDLs because they present a much larger surface area to react with oxygen and sugar.

The drawing on page 24 illustrates how you can have exactly the same amount (weight) of cholesterol in the form of pattern A and pattern B LDL, but the Bs form many more particles. So it cannot be said that all LDL is bad.

Polyunsaturated oils from seeds and grains are very easily oxidised in the blood and should be avoided at all costs – these lead to the wrong kind of cholesterol. Since there are all these different kinds of cholesterol and only the small pattern B LDLs associated with insulin resistance are atherogenic, and since it is actually pre-existing inflammation of the arteries that invites atherosclerosis, the question is: how should we check for the risk of coronary artery disease (CAD)?

The first test should be an ultra-sensitive C reactive protein (Us/CRP) test to check whether the arteries are inflamed. 'Total' cholesterol readings are pretty useless – many international medical doctors now say you should not bother with this reading. Since small, dense LDL particles, rich in triglycerides are the culprits, these should be measured to determine CAD risk. Very few pathology labs do this test so a good surrogate test is to compare HDL with triglyceride measurements and calculate the ratio of triglycerides to HDL.

To calculate the ratio of triglycerides to HDL:

If the ratio is: triglycerides divided by HDL
- 2 or less is considered ideal
- 4 = high CAD risk
- 6 = much too high

E.g. If trig = 0.79 and HDL = 1.61 then ratio = 0.49 which is excellent

In other words, the lower your triglycerides, and the higher your HDL, the smaller this ratio becomes. The Harvard-lead Boston Areas Health Study *Fasting Triglycerides, High-Density Lipoprotein, and Risk of Myocardial Infarction* reported: "High triglycerides alone increased the risk of heart attack nearly three-fold," and "the ratio of triglycerides to HDL was the strongest predictor of a heart attack, even more accurate than the LDL/HDL ratio."

HDL is measured because this is the good cholesterol, which collects fat from the tissues and transports it back to the liver. HDL is therefore protective against heart disease; so the lower the ratio, the better. A high triglyceride (fat) reading is not good, and fish oil supplementation brings triglyceride levels right down, as should avoiding sugar and following a low-carbohydrate diet.

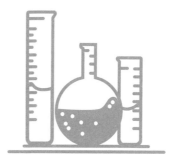

HOMOCYSTEINE.

Homocysteine should be tested, too. It is an amino acid your body makes from another amino acid called methionine, found in animal products or other protein-containing foods (including eggs, fish and sunflower seeds). This homocysteine needs to be converted to something called SAMe (S-adenosyl methionine) and glutathione, both of which have wonderful properties for the body, including prevention of depression, arthritis and liver damage.

The antioxidant glutathione is incredibly powerful and slows down the ageing process. Therefore, efficient conversion from one form to another is vitally important, but there's a catch – in order to do this, you need a long list of nutrients to be present, including magnesium, folate, zinc, TMG (trimethylglycine, which you get from choline in egg yolks), and Vitamins B2 and B12.

In order to convert homocysteine to glutathione, which is highly desirable, you will need zinc and Vitamins B2 and B12. Very often, only meat eaters have all these nutrients present to make the conversion; vegans and vegetarians can be extremely deficient in these co-factors.

When insufficiently converted, blood levels of homocysteine will rise. While the norm is anywhere between five and 15, the experts recommend that levels remain under six –

they also state that with the increase of every point, heart disease risk may rise exponentially.

There are a number of things that can go wrong if you do have a high level of homocysteine, including:

· Damage to your arteries (thickening which inhibits free circulation)
· Increased rate of ageing
· Blood has a tendency to clot more
· Lowers nitric oxide – a 'gas' which is crucial for the maintenance of healthy, flexible arteries
· A weakened immune system which is now more vulnerable to free radical damage
· Increased levels of pain and inflammation

So why do you think we hear so little about treatment for raised homocysteine levels? No drugs treat it, only nutrition and nutritional supplements will do that.

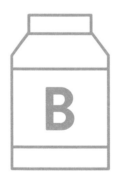

Here's how to make sure you keep your homocysteine low:

1. *Eat plenty of healthy fats and oils – on LCHF you're probably doing that already.*
2. *Eat plenty of green, leafy and colourful veggies daily.*
3. *Try not to drink more than one caffeinated drink daily.*
4. *Don't have more than one unit of alcohol daily.*
5. *Manage your stress levels.*
6. *Protein must be high quality, such as wild-caught fish, eggs, organic meats, offal and very small amounts of nuts and seeds (and no soya).*
7. *Don't even think about smoking – this is one way to raise levels significantly.*
8. *Make sure you use a mineral-rich salt like Himalayan salt (and make sure it's not the fake dyed pink salt, but the real deal).*
9. *Take a good Vitamin B Complex capsule daily in the morning at breakfast which includes folic acid.*
10. *Eat foods rich in the nutrients mentioned earlier on.*

GETTING YOUR BLOOD TESTED.

Getting your bloods done as a point of reference is a good exercise, and you should repeat the test in around six months' time, and compare them to see your progress. Here are a few you might like to ask your healthcare provider to look at for you.

HDL: This is what's known as your good cholesterol, or High Density Lipoprotein. The recommended range is 1.2 or more. However, this may be too low, so men should aim for around 1.7 or more, while women should try for as close to 2 (or a bit over) as possible. Saturated fat is one of the best ways to raise it.

LDL: This is demonised as the 'bad' cholesterol – but it's the *particle size*, not the reading, that matters. If you are off sugar and carbs, and your triglyceride count is lower than your HDL count, the likelihood is that you will have large, fluffy healthy particles, instead of small, dangerous dense low-density lipoprotein (LDL) particles. The lower your LDL goes, the more you are depriving your brain and every cell of the body of a very natural and helpful nutrient. When the LDL is too low, it has been shown the higher your cancer risk. Don't strive for low LDL, but rather for large particle size.

Triglycerides: If raised, these are synonymous with weight gain, diabetes and inflammation. A reading of 1.7 is the recommended upper limit, but around 0.5 or even less is ideal. Triglycerides are also the way the body stores fat, and the typical metabolic syndrome 'type' will have high triglycerides, low HDL and high LDL.

Lipoprotein (a) or Lp(a): This is made up of an LDL part plus a protein apoprotein (a). Elevated Lp(a) levels indicate a very strong risk factor for heart disease, as discovered by Linus Pauling. However, because this is what is called your inherited or genetic cholesterol, most doctors never test for it, as there is no drug to remedy it. Saturated fat is one way to bring this down and Vitamin C is another. Aim for a reading under 20, with 30 being borderline.

Ultrasensitive C-Reactive Protein: This is used as a marker of inflammation in your arteries, which is the true cause of heart disease.

In a nutshell, if your Us/CRP reading is:

- < 1 = indicates you have a very low risk for cardiovascular disease
- 1-3 = moderate risk
- > 3 = high risk

Homocysteine: This is an independent heart disease marker, and raised levels can thicken blood viscosity. While the recommended range is between five and 15, experts like Dr Kilmer McCully, the author of *The Homocysteine Revolution*, says it should be less than six as every point above six predisposes one to an increased CVD risk of approximately 35 per cent. All this is in reality, is a deficiency of certain B vitamins.

Fasting glucose: The normal range is 3.5 to 5.5. Because glucose will affect all the other readings, you want to have your glucose as low as possible. Being on the LCHF lifestyle should normalise this reading in time.

Fasting insulin: The reference range is between 2.1 and 10.4. You need to be as low as possible here. Raised insulin levels are inflammatory and will lead to raised Us/CRP levels as well as predispose you to a host of diseases, including obesity. Cutting carbs is a wonderful way to control insulin.

HbA1c (or glycated haemoglobin, essentially 'sugar-coated' haemoglobin): This is usually tested to determine whether or not you have diabetes and shows damage to cells over a three-month period. Ideally it should be below 5.0.

Vitamin D3: A reading of less than 30 is regarded as low. New evidence shows that levels up to 100 would be good, with the optimum range, according to experts, lying between 45 and 70. Vitamin D deficiency may affect your ability to lose weight, your pain threshold may decrease and it may possibly help prevent diabetes. It is a vital nutrient in bone building.

CONVERTING YOUR RESULTS:

If you live overseas, and wish to convert a South African test result measured in nmol/l to one measured in ng/ml, divide the nmol/l number by 2.5. For example, 50nmol/l is the same as 20ng/ml (50 ÷ 2.5). To convert a test result measured in ng/ml as we receive them here in South Africa to one measured in nmol/l, multiply the ng/ml number by 2.5. For example, 20ng/ml is the same as 50nmol/l (20 x 2.5).

PATHOLOGY

BLOOD READINGS	REFERENCE RANGE	IDEAL RANGE
HDL	> 1.2 mmol/L	> 1.7 mmol/L
LDL	< 3.0 mmol/L	3-6 mmol/L
Triglycerides	< 1.7 mmol/L	0.5-0.9 mmol/L
Lp(a)	< 30 mmol/L	< 20 mmol/L
Us/CRP	1-3 mg/L	< 1 mg/L
Homocysteine	5-15 umol/L	< 6 umol/L
Glucose	3.5-5.5 mmol/L	same
Insulin	2.1-10.4 mIU/L	< 5.5 mIU/L
HbA1c	< 5.5%	< 5.5%
Vitamin D3	> 30 ng/mL	> 45 ng/mL
T4	7.2-16.4 pmol/L	same
T3	3.8-6.0 pmol/L	same
TSH	0.37-3.5 mIU/L	0.37-2.0 mIU/L
Thyroglobulin AB	0-4 IU/L	same
Thyroid peroxidase AB	0-9 IU/L	same

These last five readings tell you what is going on with your thyroid gland (see the thyroid section) and for you to compare your blood results. Some people respond quickly, others take much longer. Be aware that your LDL *may* go up and take up to a year to settle – this is not dangerous; it is merely adjusting the size of the particles. LDL is not dangerous or 'bad' – it's just another part of the equation. A healthy body will automatically stabilise in time. As we age, we are *supposed* to have higher cholesterol – so bear that in mind.

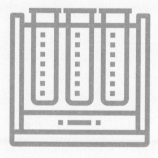

Chapter

01

BACK TO BASICS: MACRONUTRIENTS

The human diet consists of three macronutrients: protein, fat and carbohydrates. Two of these are essential to life: protein and fat. We have no need for carbohydrates as the body is able to generate these from protein and fat as needed. However, we do need to eat vegetables, which have a mixture of these three macronutrients. Therefore, when we eat vegetables, we automatically eat some carbohydrates. This includes fibre, which is also a carbohydrate. Fibre does not significantly raise blood sugar, so we can deduct it from the total carb count to get a net carb count. Micronutrients found in vegetables (such as vitamins, minerals and phytonutrients) act as co-factors for the metabolism of the macronutrients in the cell and are a healthy part of any diet.

CARBOHYDRATES.

Carbohydrates are found in all food except fat and animal protein. They comprise mainly sugars, which are called simple carbohydrates, starches and grains, which are often referred to as complex carbohydrates, and fibre. Carbs elicit a much faster spike in glucose than the other two macronutrients and, while fibre is not digested as such, it does have beneficial health properties.

It's now believed a high-carbohydrate diet may cause heart disease, Alzheimer's disease, cancer and many other health conditions. While carbohydrates are restricted on this lifestyle, most vegetables, in particular green vegetables grown above ground, are encouraged as part of a healthy diet. There are no essential carbohydrates, nor essential sugars, but fat and protein are both essential.

FAT.

Fat is an essential nutrient for the human body – without fat you'd die. It is an energy source (like petrol to a car), a building block for hormones and provides satiety. Food is more flavourful with fat, without which one would start craving sugar as an alternative source of flavour. There is saturated fat which you need not fear; polyunsaturated fat, which we don't want in an unnatural form, as in seed oils; and monounsaturated fat, as found in foods like olives and avocado. All fat is made up of all three of these fats – it's just the different ratio of saturated to polyunsaturated to monounsaturated that determines the type of fat.

PROTEIN.

Protein is essential to life. It is made up of amino acids; a 'complete' protein will have all 22 common amino acids, nine of which are essential for adults and another four for children and infants. The alphabet is made up of 26 letters, now imagine the 'alphabet' of a complete protein – this alphabet has 22 amino acids instead of letters, which are building blocks. From just 26 letters we form every word we have in the English language, and in the same way we form every kind of protein from these 22 amino acids (over 50,000). In each case it's the sequence and length that makes the difference.

Only nine of these amino acids are essential. The others can be manufactured from these; they are the raw materials. When you eat animal flesh, you get all nine essential ones – and most of the others too, unlike vegans. You may recognise some names of proteins: milk has casein and whey, whereas red meat has collagen, actin and myosin.

Plant proteins have different names but none of them are complete proteins as you find in the animal kingdom, as they all lack some of the nine essential amino acid building blocks.

Chapter

02

CLARIFYING THE CREED

The doctor of the future will give no medicine, but will interest his patients in the care of the human frame, in diet and in the cause and prevention of disease.

– Thomas A Edison

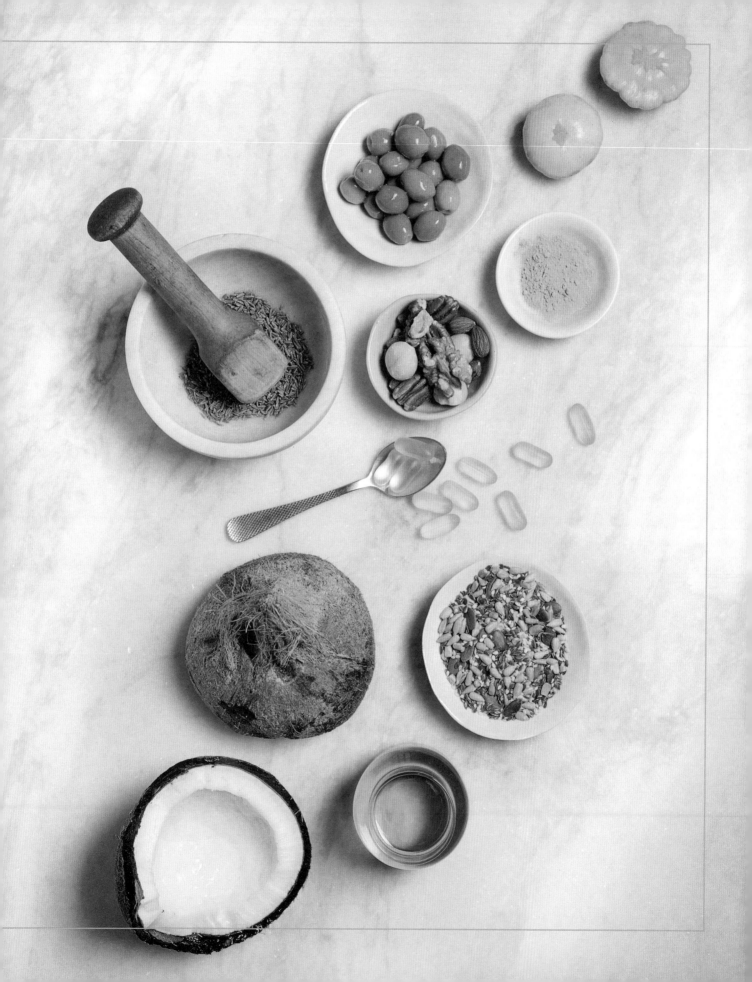

Chapter

02

FATS AND OILS

How did we get to the point of being so terribly afraid of fat? To cut a long story short: in the 1970s, saturated fat was demonised as dangerous thanks to one Ancel Keys, an American scientist who falsified evidence to mislead an expert panel. To this day, his 'findings' are revered as the gold standard throughout most of the Western world. Essentially, without any real proof or proper scientific research, the decision was taken to roll out the low-fat lie that is accepted as conventional wisdom. The world has tragically followed it ever since, with devastating consequences.

Fat intake worldwide has decreased, while gym membership is through the roof – and so is the rate of obesity, Alzheimer's, dementia, cancer, heart disease and diabetes. Saturated fat is clearly not to blame.

One of society's main misconceptions about healthy fat is that it causes weight gain and that it is bad for the heart. To say this is unscientific is putting it mildly – healthy fat has been shown to have nothing to do with heart disease and rather than causing weight gain, it can often greatly assist with weight loss.

In 2014, Sweden became the first Western nation to develop national dietary guidelines rejecting the popular low-fat diet dogma in favour of a low-carb high-fat diet. Based on a review of 16,000 studies, the prominent Swedish Agency for Health Technology Assessment and Assessment of Social Services (SBU) said the best foods for losing weight are high-fat ones, which include olive and coconut oils. A recent study from the SBU health committee recommended a low-carb diet for weight loss. A keen advocate of saturated fat since 2006, Professor Fredrik Nyström stated in an article in the Swedish paper *Corren* that there was no reason to be concerned about any danger or harm that could be associated with these fats. The LCHF diet is finally being accepted into the mainstream and the fear of fat no longer holds water.

A LCHF diet has been shown to increase HDL levels (high density lipoproteins) without any adverse effects on LDL (low density lipoproteins). This applies to both a moderate low-carbohydrate intake of less than 40 per cent of the total energy intake, as well as to the stricter low-carbohydrate diet, where carbohydrate intake is less than 20 per cent of the total energy intake. In addition, the stricter low-carbohydrate diet seems to greatly improve glucose levels for individuals with obesity and diabetes, and lowers dangerously high triglyceride levels.

The Swedish council found that butter, olive oil, double cream and bacon are not harmful foods – quite the opposite. Fat, they said, is the best thing for those who wish to lose weight, and a high-fat diet doesn't cause cardiovascular disease. Low-fat diets lack solid scientific basis. Nyström's report turns what we have been taught on its head and advocates a low-carbohydrate, high-fat diet as being the most effective weapon against obesity.

Nyström states: "I've been working with this for so long. It feels great to have this scientific report, and that the scepticism towards low-carb diets among my colleagues has disappeared during the course of the work. When all recent scientific studies are lined up the result is indisputable: our deep-seated fear of fat is completely unfounded. You don't get fat from fatty foods, just as you don't get atherosclerosis from calcium or turn green from green vegetables."

By restricting carbohydrate-rich foods high in sugar and starch, one can achieve healthy levels of insulin, blood lipids and HDL cholesterol. This means eliminating sugar, potatoes and grains from the diet and embracing olive oil, butter, oily fish and fattier meat cuts. "If you eat potatoes you might as well eat candy," says Nyström.

"Potatoes contain glucose units in a chain, which is converted to sugar in the GI tract. Such a diet causes blood sugar, and then the hormone insulin, to skyrocket."

SATURATED FAT.

Saturated fat is absolutely essential in the human diet. Membranes are formed by important phospholipids in every cell made up mostly of saturated fatty acids, particularly in the brain where more than 80 per cent of the phospholipids carry half of their fatty acids as saturated. The lungs have a very high need for saturated fats – lung surfactant is a very important class of phospholipid made up of 100 per cent saturated fatty acids called dipalmitoylphosphatidylcholine. When you eat hydrogenated fats and oils, these damaged fats get used by the lungs which will not function as effectively.

New research suggests that the trans-fatty acids found in these unnatural fats are causing asthma in children. Fat gives taste, satiety, pleasure and decreases the desire for sweet things, addictive foods and triggers pleasure receptors in the brain. Without fats, you won't absorb your all-important fat-soluble Vitamins A, D, E and K.

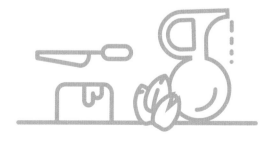

WHY SEED OILS ARE NOT LCHF.

It needs to be said: seed oils of any kind are not LCHF nor Paleo – nor healthy for that matter. Seed oils are notoriously unstable. In order to promote shelf life, they have been subjected to very high heat and are therefore damaged trans fats and as such, are highly inflammatory to the human body. Even the cold-pressed ones are unstable and go rancid quickly. The ratio of omega-6 to omega-3 fats is also a deciding factor – excessive amounts of omega-6 present in these oils cause rampant widespread inflammation, resulting in disease states. Polyunsaturated fats contribute to insulin resistance. Like sugar, seed oils are an unnatural food owing to the effects of processing.

If you wish to use high monounsaturated oil, extra virgin olive oil is still the best choice due to the limited processing techniques used. In addition, it has been around for thousands of years – we don't yet know the full implications of any new, possibly genetically altered oil. The LCHF lifestyle bans all seed and grain oils out of hand, no matter what their claims may be. Olive oil, macadamia oil and avocado oils are about the only ones safe to

STEERING CLEAR OF SEED OILS

- Cheap, damaged oils make us sick; these are no replacement for 'real' food.
- Our bodies battle to metabolise these as they are unnatural.
- They place the pancreas, liver and entire digestive system under severe strain.
- They are highly inflammatory – they may cause cardiovascular disease and other diseases by inflaming arteries.
- They may prevent weight loss and could foster weight gain.
- They displace protective omega-3 fats due to high inflammatory omega-6 fatty acid levels.

- They have been shown to cause cancer.
- There is no scientific evidence whatsoever that they are healthy – the converse is true.
- They are prohibited for use in infant formula as it retards growth (discovered by the FDA in 1985).
- Synthetic and harmful antioxidants are used to prevent them from going rancid (e.g. butylated hydroxytoluene or BHT) to compensate for the loss of antioxidants – these have been shown to be carcinogenic.

use. As these are fruit and nut oils, they are more stable and have a much longer natural shelf life, so don't need processing.

David Gillespie's bestseller, *Toxic Oil*, exposes the way in which vegetable oils cause cancer, heart disease, eye damage and harm the immune system. His book, *Big Fat Lies: How the Industry is Making You Sick, Fat and Poor*, begins with these words: "'Vegetable' oil makes you exceedingly vulnerable to cancer. Every extra mouthful of vegetable oil you consume takes you one step closer to a deadly (and irreversible) outcome." Strong words, but it seems we need to be shocked to stop us believing that these oils are benign or even healthy. In 2013, the *Canadian Medical Association Journal* confirmed that these oils raise the risk of heart disease and suggested Canadian health authorities reconsider cholesterol-lowering claims on foods containing vegetable oils.

BRINGING BALANCE.

Think of omega-3 and omega-6 as being at either end of a see-saw. When one is down, the other is up – we want them balanced at a 1:1 ratio.

The ratio in Western society now is around 20:1. The correct ratio of omega-6 to omega-3 is critical as imbalance leads to diseases of inflammation like asthma, hypertension, digestive disturbances, depressed immunity, weight gain, sterility and maybe cancer. While omega-6 is an essential fatty acid, as is omega-3, we get too much omega-6 in our diet and not enough omega-3. It's ultimately omega-3 (from fish oil and fatty fish) that we are short of.

An important paper by the late Professor Mary Enig and Sally Fallon, *The Oiling of America*, is a must-read if you really want to understand the full impact of polyunsaturated fats on our health. Vegetable oils are subject to rancidity, increasing the body's need for antioxidants; they cause damage to reproductive organs and lungs, interfere with cognitive function and learning ability, are liver-toxic, harmful to the immune system, suppress infant growth mentally and physically, increase levels of uric acid in the blood, accelerate ageing, and they increase the risk of cancer, cardiovascular disease, weight gain and autoimmune disease. There is absolutely nothing healthy about them. The best way to balance your omega-6 to omega-3 ratio is to eat unprocessed, single-ingredient foods (from which you will get plenty of omega-6), and eat wild-caught fatty fish, free-range eggs, free-range meat, unsprayed vegetables and other high-quality sources of food.

Vegetable oils will often have two rather nasty substances present: butylated hydroxyanisole (BHA) and BHT. These are artificial antioxidants which prolong shelf life, but have also been shown to create potential cancer-causing compounds in the body. They have been linked to conditions such as immune system irregularities, infertility, behavioural problems, liver and kidney damage and weight gain.

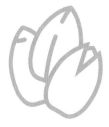

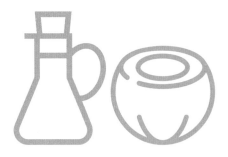

All fats and oils have different percentages of saturated fat, monounsaturated fat and polyunsaturated fat. The proportions of these three fats give the fat/oil the classification of saturated, monounsaturated or polyunsaturated. Saturated fats are extremely stable even at very high temperatures, but polyunsaturated fatty acids become particularly harmful to health when heated due to the free radicals and trans fats formed. Monounsaturated fats are somewhere in the middle.

Polyunsaturated fatty acids, which are liquid at room temperature, can be made solid (as in margarine). Hydrogen is added at high temperatures to achieve this. Polyunsaturated fats are already harmful to begin with, and hydrogenation is an added health concern.

VEGETABLE OILS.

Have you ever seen a vegetable dripping with oil? Of course not, there's no such thing. The rising rates of cancer, obesity, diabetes, heart disease, Alzheimer's disease and every other disease tell us that our switch to these unnatural, man-made chemical substances has had the opposite effect to what they promise. They've created an epidemic of ill health.

Our grandparents used fat found in nature – lard, butter, ghee, duck fat, goose fat and bacon fat – yet we've been brainwashed into thinking that they will kill us.

Vegetable oils don't come from vegetables; they come from genetically modified seeds (usually) like rapeseed (canola), soyabean, corn, sunflower, safflower, peanut and cottonseed. The extraction process is completely unnatural and carried out under extreme temperatures with the use of dangerous chemicals, solvents and even heavy metals to increase yield. They are cheap and hazardous substitutes for the real thing because the processing has caused the *cis* bond to become a *trans* bond – changing the structure of the fat and making it unnatural.

Processed food is laced with these dangerous fats, and even good restaurants use them as they are cheap and tasteless. The contrast between these fake fats and real butter is phenomenal. Making butter is a very simple process: cream is separated from milk, shaken or churned, and in a short time you have butter. Compare this with seed oils, which go through a rigorous process where they are heated to alarmingly high temperatures, combined with petroleum solvents to extract the oil, and re-heated again. Acid is then added to remove wax solids formed during the first processing. More chemicals are put into the mix to improve the colour and the oil which then has to be deodorised in order to remove the chemical processing smell. If you hydrogenate this now, you get margarine. And to top it all, it tastes so ghastly they have had to remove the taste and replace it with a buttery taste in the form of a carcinogenic chemical called diacetyl. If you want butter flavour, just eat butter.

Because these fats and oils are so unstable, they oxidise very quickly and easily. This oxidation causes inflammation and mutation in cells. It's no wonder we have cancer, heart disease, endometriosis, PCOS and other inflammatory diseases running riot in our society – these oils inflame. Nina Teicholz's excellent book, *Big Fat Surprise*, is essential reading for anyone who still thinks fat is the enemy.

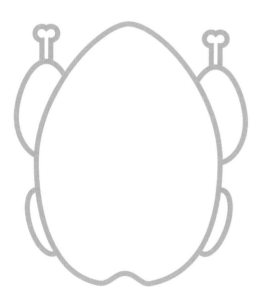

PRACTICAL TIPS FOR AVOIDING POLYUNSATURATED FAT.

- *Never buy 'oil blends' – blended oils are usually damaged, cheap and unhealthy.*
- *Avoid all seed and grain oils as a matter of course – use coconut, olive, macadamia and avocado oil if you wish to use liquid oil.*
- *Never buy oil in plastic – we believe all fats and oils should only be sold in glass, never plastic.*
- *Butter is healthy, margarine is not.*
- *Avoid deep-fried foods unless fried in virgin coconut oil or lard.*
- *Never eat anything made with hydrogenated oils (onion rings, chips, deep-fried food).*
- *Only buy raw or activated nuts, never roasted, they are usually deep fried in damaged oils.*
- *Enjoy natural sources of fat from foods such as avocado, nuts and seeds, wild-caught fish, organic eggs, chicken and meats, coconut milk and raw olive oil.*

Don't be afraid of healthy fat, but do be afraid of unhealthy vegetable oils – be very afraid. A study showed that even a two per cent increase in trans fats has been associated with a 23 per cent increased risk in cardiovascular disease.

The elephant in the room whenever there is discussion around fats and oils is the issue of cholesterol. By now, most people in the LCHF movement know that cholesterol is a natural substance made by the liver to protect us, not kill us.

We also know cholesterol is there to:

· Make hormones
· Give strength and rigidity to cell membranes
· Make Vitamin D (vital for bones, nervous system, muscle tone, immunity and growth)
· Produce bile for fat digestion
· Act as an antioxidant to protect against cellular damage, which causes cancer and heart disease
· Maintain a healthy intestinal lining
· Repair damaged blood vessels

The consumption of vegetable oils and margarine has increased 400 per cent, while the consumption of sugar and processed food has increased by 60 per cent. From 1910 to 1970, the average intake of butter in the United States dropped from 18 kilograms a year to 1.8 kilograms a year, according to an article for the Weston A Price Foundation. It's all back to front.

It's not difficult to replace damaged fats with healthy ones, and they taste so much better. Virtually all processed food and condiments will contain one or more unhealthy oils. Just eat real food and make it yourself. An occasional night out is not the end of the world, but choose your restaurant carefully, where quality food is served and good oils are used.

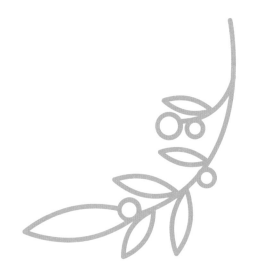

DAMAGED/UNSTABLE OILS TO BE AVOIDED

- **Canola oil:** Over 80 per cent of the canola grown in the United States is genetically modified and although no GM crops are grown commercially in the UK, they can be imported. High in inflammatory omega-6, they damage the body.
- **Corn oil:** Just as bad as the rest, and it is shown to cause liver damage – besides, it's a grain oil.
- **Cottonseed oil:** Worst of all oils, this is full of pesticides (cotton is the most heavily sprayed crop on the planet). It is highly carcinogenic, and often added to oil blends.
- **Flaxseed oil:** This is unstable and unable to be converted to anti-inflammatory omega-3 DHA and EPA, which is the reason for taking it in the first place.
- **Grapeseed oil:** Don't be misled by the high smoke point – oils with higher smoke points may be important to a chef, but they have nothing to do with health benefits or safety. If the oil is classed as polyunsaturated, you should not cook with it, irrespective of its smoke point. Grapeseed oil is predominantly classified as a polyunsaturated fatty acid, and is thus highly reactive. Free radical production quickly takes place when these fatty acids are exposed to any degree of heat, even very low heat. You need to see this as a red flag for producing inflammation and irritation within your body – grapeseed oil is a whopping 71 per cent polyunsaturated fat.
- **Margarines:** These are man-made products from seed oils that are usually partially hydrogenated.
- **Soyabean oil:** This is a close second to cottonseed, and widely used in the restaurant, fast-food and processed food industries. Most products that profess to use 'vegetable' oil are using soyabean oil, which is harmful, inflammatory, genetically modified and carcinogenic – damaging to the body.
- **Sunflower, safflower oils:** These and all the other 'baddies' are just as dangerous – damaged, devoid of any health-giving properties, they cause inflammation and disease.
- **'Vegetable' oils:** Oils like peanut, soya, corn, and cottonseed oils are unstable and extremely harmful.

Note: Did you know that just 50 years ago paint and varnishes were made using soyabean oil, safflower oil and linseed (flaxseed) oil? They were never meant for eating, but for industry. Once they learnt how to make paint from petrol, they turned their attention to using the seeds for human consumption – and the rest is history.

FATS AND OILS FOR COOKING.

Butter and ghee

Who doesn't love butter? It has incredible flavour and is nutritious. Ghee is clarified butter and a good choice; it's also easy to make yourself.

There is so much misguided information about butter. People have been eating butter forever – and they weren't dropping dead of heart attacks and strokes. Butter even used to be thought of as medicinal, which it is, due to it containing Vitamins K2 and D, and only became 'unhealthy' when big business developed margarine.

Lard and tallow

Lard is rendered pork fat, while tallow is rendered beef or mutton fat. Both are excellent solid cooking fats, very stable over high heat and perfect for higher temperature frying. Lard is particularly good because it has a neutral flavour, so for recipes where you don't really want to taste the fat, this is a great option. I need to emphasise that when you're cooking with animal fats, you really do want to get them from grass-fed, pastured animals that haven't been injected with hormones and antibiotics.

Olive oil

A truly excellent oil, and a relatively stable one full of wonderful polyphenols. There are basically three types of olive oil: extra virgin, virgin, and pure. Extra virgin is a range of oil in the top grade from the first pressing of the olives, as is virgin olive oil.

The difference lies with the acidity level of the oil. Better oils have less acidity and stronger flavours. After those two, you have a range of 'pure' oils, which are typically refined in some way and definitely best avoided. Extra virgin organic olive oil in a dark glass bottle is our strong recommendation.

Coconut oil

A marvellous oil, usually having a slight coconut flavour, and excellent for high-temperature cooking. It goes so well with so many types of sauce, especially those with a little sweetness.

Coconut oil has had a bad rap in the past couple of decades because it's saturated. The type of saturated fat in coconut oil, known as medium-chain triglycerides, has been proven to be supremely healthy. It is shelf-stable and heat-stable, and will remain stable and delicious in your pantry for ages without issues. And by the way, it helps weight loss. Just saying...

Duck fat and fatty cuts of meat

These are all healthy, natural fats. Enjoy them. Keep coconut oil, butter, ghee, lard, duck fat and olive oil in your kitchen – it's really all you need.

For extra flavour, there are some nut oils that you can try, like walnut oil, almond oil and hazelnut oil. Nut oils are fine if properly pressed, as they are stable.

SUMMARY:
GOOD AND BAD/UNSTABLE
COOKING FATS

GOOD FATS	BAD AND UNSTABLE FATS
Coconut (organic)	Canola oil
Palm oil (only red, sustainably sourced)	Hydrogenated palm oil
Butter, ghee	Corn oil
Lard (from pigs)	Cottonseed oil
Schmaltz (chicken fat)	Vegetable blend oils
Tallow (beef or lamb fat)	Soyabean oil
Duck fat	Sunflower oil (all kinds)
Full fat dairy (if not intolerant)	Rice bran oil
Fat on pastured meats	Margarine and shortening
Olive oil	Butter 'spreads' (as opposed to pure butter)
Avocado oil	Partially hydrogenated fats and oils
Macadamia nut oil	Flaxseed oil
Pecan oil, walnut oil	Trans fats

FISH OIL.

Science has clearly shown the benefits of fish oil in well over 3,000 impressive scientific studies. A US National Institutes of Health study published in the *Journal of Lipid Research* shows that none of the alpha-linolenic acid (ALA) in flax oil can convert into docosahexaenoic acid (DHA) and only two per cent can convert into eicosapentaenoic acid (EPA). The scientists concluded that flaxseed oil is not a viable source of omega-3 in the diet.

Omega-3 fish oil benefits your health in an enormous way. From your brain, to your heart, to every joint in every part of the body – and everywhere else in-between – fish oil can vastly improve the quality of your life. The omega-3 fish oil fatty acids EPA and DHA occur naturally in fish oil and are necessary for healthy conception, pregnancy and lactation. Production of fertile eggs and sperm, plus optimum growth and development of the foetus are all dependent on omega-3.

Studies published in the **American Journal of Clinical Nutrition** *show that fish oils:*

- *Lower bad cholesterol*
- *Lower triglycerides*
- *Lower blood pressure*
- *Prevent and reduce painful inflammatory illnesses (arthritis, asthma, colitis)*

Other omega-3 fish oil benefits include significantly lowering your risk of:

- *Stroke*
- *Diabetes*
- *Depression*
- *Heart disease*
- *Certain cancers*
- *Arthritis*
- *Sudden cardiac death*

The best omega-3 fatty acids, DHA and EPA sources are salmon, tuna, sardines, anchovies and herring. These omega-3 fatty acids are not found in lean fish, such as cod or halibut, or lean non-cold water fish, only fatty, deep water fish.

Fish oil, in fish or in a supplement, is incredibly valuable in protecting against a host of chronic disease conditions – and even the seemingly not-so-important ones. The trouble is, if you suffer from these 'unimportant' ones, like eczema or dry skin, you may not be concerned, but internally you are deficient too, and the results of that deficiency could be far-reaching.

PROBLEMS ASSOCIATED WITH TOO MUCH DIETARY OMEGA-6 FAT

* You could be ageing prematurely.
* Cancer may be connected with excess omega-6 oils due to their inflammatory nature.
* Your triglycerides may climb and your healthy HDL level may fall.
* Your insulin sensitivity may be compromised, so you could have high levels of insulin.

It is important to increase omega-3 levels and maintain lower levels of omega-6. Try following these steps:

* Take fish oil daily, or eat fatty fish three times a week.
* Do not buy or take supplements containing omega-6 or omega-9. You're already awash with omega-6, and your body readily makes its own omega-9. It's not an 'essential' fatty acid.
* Avoid all fizzy and sugary drinks. These raise insulin, cause weight gain, inflame your body and create all the conditions you are trying to avoid, including insulin resistance.
* Avoid cooking with grain and seed oils, they are flooded with damaged omega-6 fats.
* Avoid all grains and their brans (often sold as fibre replacements).

FLAXSEED OIL VERSUS FISH OIL.

Many people take flaxseed oil thinking it's healthy. The hype around it is as much a deception in the health industry as statins are in the medical arena. It seems it is neither necessary nor healthy. Flaxseed oil is, after all, a seed oil, and LCHF does not include seed oils at all.

In a nutshell, alpha-linolenic acid (ALA), the kind of omega-3 long-chain fatty acid found in flaxseed oil, cannot be efficiently converted into the DHA and EPA your body needs – and the prime reason for taking omega-3 oil in the first place is to be able to execute that conversion. It just doesn't happen. ALA does not have the same benefits as the long-chain fatty acids DHA and EPA. Flaxseed oil is also very high in omega-6, an inflammatory fat; while the omega-3 it boasts is actually just ALA, not DHA or EPA.

Our food is awash with omega-6. Nuts and a few seeds will give you ALA, so there is no need to gulp it down in oil. Flaxseed oil may cause men to grow breasts, and there is some evidence it may contribute to prostate cancer and fertility problems owing to its phytoestrogenic effect. Eating seeds in moderation is fine though.

COULD YOU HAVE AN ESSENTIAL FATTY ACID DEFICIENCY?

Answer yes or no to the following symptoms. If you have been consuming too many seed oils, you can expect the answer to be yes even before you begin.

- Accelerated ageing
- Acne
- Aggression
- Allergies
- Alligator skin (rough and hard)
- Arthritis
- Brittle, easily frayed fingernails which split
- 'Chicken skin' on back of arms
- Cracked skin on heels or fingertips
- Compromised immunity and/or kidney function
- Difficulty concentrating
- Depression and anxiety
- Dry eyes
- Dry skin and hair
- Dry, unmanageable hair
- Digestive problems
- Excessive thirst
- Fatigue
- Frequent infections
- Frequent urination
- Hyperactivity
- Irritability
- Joint pain
- Learning and memory problems
- Lowered immunity
- Patches of pale skin on cheeks
- Poor wound healing
- Soft nails

If you find you have answered yes to more than five symptoms, there is a strong possibility you may be deficient. A good-quality, pharmaceutical-grade fish oil is helpful at around three grams a day. Please use a good quality oil for best results and exclude all supplemental omega-6 sources as it would automatically mean an excess of omega-6 in the diet. Too much omega-6 always means too little omega-3. The benefits of using fish oil are remarkable, ranging from heart health to brain health; it's probably the most studied nutrient in history and boasts thousands of health benefits.

KRILL OIL
VERSUS FISH OIL

Krill oil is beneficial and certainly better than any plant-based oil. However, it is not a viable alternative to omega-3 fish oil for a number of reasons:

- The level of DHA is extremely low at only nine per cent compared to over 40 per cent in fish oil.
- It is no purer than fish oil because of the purifying process used in pharmaceutical grade or ultra-refined fish oil. Very small fish are used for good fish oil, which have virtually no contaminants – all of which are removed by molecular distillation.
- Its bioavailability is not considered scientifically superior; fish and krill oil are believed to be completely on a par with one another in this respect.
- It is more expensive than good omega-3 oil from fish.
- Sadly, by harvesting krill we are denuding the oceans of the start of the entire food chain.
- We would not naturally consume krill, but we would eat fish.

Fish oil has 200 per cent more DHA, and 600 to 800 per cent more EPA gram for gram than krill, and all beneficial studies on omega-3 have been done using fish oil. As yet, there are no long-term studies on krill, so maybe wait a few years to see if this trend lasts. At the time of writing it is not eco-certified to my knowledge. Krill is the primary food source for penguins and whales; and harvesting it may be raping our oceans of their source of food.

Chapter

02

PROTEIN POWER

Because of the enormous importance of protein in the diet, it needs to be covered more fully. However, please remember a low-carb lifestyle will promote:

· Low-carbohydrate intake
· More fat than you were used to on the now-defunct, low-fat diet – but it's healthy fat
· Moderate protein intake from animal sources. This is not a high-protein lifestyle

In order to understand the role of protein, you need to understand exactly what protein consists of, and what it actually does. Let's look at it very simply. Think of protein as a little house made of bricks. Protein is the *whole* house, but the bricks are called amino acids. If you build a house of these bricks, it is then called a protein; but if you build it from wood and stones, and a couple of bricks all over the place, you could say it's no longer a solid house but more of an unfinished garden shed. Animal protein then is the house, not the shed. Plant protein can be said to be the shed in that it has some bricks, but very few, the rest are not materials that provide a solid structure.

Animal protein has amino acid bricks, and as a complete protein it's comprised of nine essential amino acid 'bricks', various non-essential amino acids and even some conditional ones. The essential ones are vital to make up this complete protein because the others can in fact be made from nine essential 'bricks'.

Protein plays a major role in the body, with hundreds of functions: repair, the production of hormones, digestive enzymes, energy, prevention of muscle wasting, immunity, the production of enzymes – there isn't one cell which does not require protein.

Vegans and vegetarians may eventually suffer from nutritional deficiency symptoms so we do not recommend this lifestyle. It's also virtually impossible to be LCHF and vegan as it is a high-carb lifestyle by default. Protein is crucial to life – our bodies cannot repair themselves without it.

HOW MUCH PROTEIN DO YOU *NEED*?

This is highly individual, depending on whether you are athletic, sedentary, old, young, sick or well. The most common method used to estimate daily protein requirement is to multiply your body weight in kilograms by 0.8 as your minimum intake, although you can have more if you are athletic, pregnant or elderly, or simply feel you need more. Studies have shown that obese people who eat at least 30 per cent protein (around 56 grams daily) preserve muscle mass far more successfully. Those who under-eat (around 18 per cent of protein) actually lose lean muscle mass as well as fat – quite an incentive not to under-eat protein.

Say you are sedentary and weigh 55 kilograms – you would need between 44 to 95 grams of protein daily. (NB: This is complete protein as found in animal products, not vegetarian protein which doesn't contain all nine essential amino acids). It's virtually impossible to meet your protein requirements if you are vegetarian or vegan. Athletes need to calculate one to two grams protein daily for each kilogram of body weight. More protein is needed when you are injured, as protein is required for repair – so 1.5`grams protein per kilogram is needed here, but make sure it's good quality protein. Elderly people lose thigh muscle mass very quickly when given just the typical 0.8 grams protein per kilogram. They need more.

PROTEIN 101.

If you overdo protein (very high protein), you may suffer from bad breath, so rather eat more fat and less protein. To guide you: 28 grams of meat or fish has approximately seven grams of protein if cooked, and six grams if raw. In order to know how much food you need to consume to take in the protein you need, consult the helpful list on page 50.

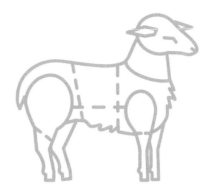

ANIMAL ORGANS.

Organ meats and offal are making a comeback. They are the most healthful part of the animal. When a predatory mammal kills its prey, it goes straight for the organs, and leaves the muscle meat for the other scavengers.

Organ meats are rich in nutrients while being relatively inexpensive, due to lack of demand. They usually end up in processed meats or dog food, and while they were used extensively in cooking a few decades ago, they became a forgotten source of high-quality nourishment.

It doesn't help that organ meats are demonised for having fat and cholesterol, which is such a shame. Our grandparents knew the worth of organ meats and placed great value on liver, heart and kidneys, using these foods to support the health of their own organs. We can do the same, and you will find some recipes for forgotten parts of the animal in this book.

GRAMS OF PROTEIN IN ANIMAL FOODS

ANIMAL FOOD	PORTION	PROTEIN
Beef mince (patty)	112g	28g
Steak	168g	42g
Most cuts of beef	28g	7g
Chicken breast	100g	30g
Chicken thigh	1	10g
Chicken drumstick	1	11g
Chicken wing	1	6g
Cooked chicken	112g	35g
Fish fillets	100g	22g
Tuna	168g	40g
Pork chop	1	22g
Pork loin or tenderloin	112g	29g
Pork mince (raw)	28g	5g
Pork mince (cooked)	84g	22g
Bacon	Large slice or 5 rashers	3g
Egg	1	6-7g
Milk	1 cup	8g
Cottage cheese	½ cup	15g
Yoghurt	1 cup	8-12g
Soft cheeses (Brie)	28g	6g
Medium cheeses (Cheddar)	28g	7-8g
Hard cheeses (Parmesan)	28g	10g

You need a moderate amount of protein (usually around the size your palm). Clearly, this does not mean half a chicken for lunch and a T-bone steak every night. Eat animal fat, and eat the internal organs of the animal too (called nose-to-tail eating). Buy fatty cuts of meat and eat the fat from lamb, steaks, chicken skin and chops. Please also use the pan juices – don't waste a drop.

If you can locate produce that is 'clean' and humanely reared without hormones and steroids, you are doing really well. Animals caringly raised without chemicals and poor quality grain-based feed (like soya and corn) and humanely slaughtered provide the best quality food. You will also find that you won't eat as much when the quality is good as it's far more nutritious, and you'll feel satisfied sooner.

Search through old cookbooks from decades ago and you'll find literally hundreds of recipes for all sorts of organ meats. Liver was considered a staple of the diet; it was sautéed, used in dumplings and pastries, eaten raw, puréed, roasted and minced. When hunters killed an animal, it was tradition to eat the raw warm liver on the spot, with everyone in the hunting party having a share. This was not only a tradition among European hunters, but was also practised by the Native Americans and other indigenous people. There are hundreds of traditional European sausages made from liver, liverwurst being just one of them. Pâtés are one of the tastiest results of this tradition.

There were myriad recipes containing kidneys, heart, brains, sweetbreads (thymus gland), intestines, even lungs, spleens and other organs. These organs were made into sausages, pies, soups, fritters, and preparations unique to each organ. It was traditional to stuff the stomach of an animal with chopped organ meat and other foods, and the famous Scottish Haggis is an example of this practice. Most of these recipes required a great deal of work, because the majority of organ meats require a lot of trimming. There are often membranes, veins, arteries, and other inedible parts that must be removed. The edible portions usually require soaking, often multiple soakings, pounding, and intense cleaning. These recipes frequently went into great detail.

The healthy cultures studied by the well-known dentist, Dr Weston A Price, all ate organ meats and valued them highly. Their traditional preparations of these meats involved a great deal of work in cleaning and preparing the organs. It should be noted that many of these dishes did not taste particularly good and were resisted by children. People ate them anyway, and forced their children to eat them. Why did they go to all that work and trouble? Because they knew there was something in these organ meats that was good for them, and because this knowledge had been handed down from generation to generation.

It's so sad that when you tell people to eat organ meats today, a look of horror crosses their faces. We've forgotten how to eat and prepare these nutrient-rich foods, but we need to do so due to the enormous benefits they offer.

The organ meat of factory animals is not the same as that which has been eaten for thousands of years, as the animals have usually been given hormones and antibiotics, and have not been fed their natural feed.

A preferred way to eat organ meat is in the form of sausages, made by a good butcher. Great care must be taken in choosing sausage, because all kinds of undesirable ingredients are often added to them. Insist on knowing everything that is in a sausage before you eat it. A delicious liverwurst could contain liver, heart and kidney, and perhaps some spices. You can also make pâté and liver loaves. Organ meats are some of the most vital and nutrient-dense foods available.

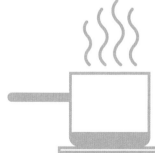

Chapter

02

SCARY SUGAR

An entire slave trade was built on it, and it is seductively introduced into almost every food on the shelves. However, the removal of sugar from the diet is a pivotal part of LCHF, Paleo and proper low carb real food living. While some say sugar is as addictive as cocaine, there is no medical evidence to support this theory. You can easily stop sugar without medical intervention or life-threatening withdrawal, unlike some drugs. Technically, eating sugar is not an addiction, yet there is a psychological addiction, if you like, that does seem to grab people. The only way to beat it is by following the LCHF lifestyle. Protein and fat are the two crutches you will need as you give up this dangerous substance.

WHAT HAPPENS WHEN YOU EAT SUGAR.

Carbohydrates in any form, particularly grains and table sugar, are seen by the body as sugar as they are converted very quickly into glucose, and will cause a blood sugar spike. Eating carbs causes the pancreas to release the hormone insulin to reduce that spike. Insulin regulates the level of sugar in the blood – the more sugar in the bloodstream, the more insulin is released. Insulin then goes on to store glucose in the liver and muscles in the form of glycogen and fat. If too much insulin is released, your blood sugar will drop too low, causing low blood sugar. This causes you to crave carbs, and the vicious cycle begins again.

DID YOU KNOW?

- In the 1800s, people consumed **1.3 teaspoons of sugar a day.**
- In 2012, Americans consumed **38 teaspoons** of sugar every five days, or 58 kilograms of sugar a year. (That's the size of some people.) Now, the figure is no doubt higher.

When you eat sugar your body can deal with it in one of two ways:

1. **Burn it for energy** if your body has a healthy metabolism.
2. **Convert it to fat and store it in your fat cells**. Today most people are stressed, lead a sedentary lifestyle and have an extremely poor diet, which causes fat storage.

Every time you have more sugar or carbs, you set this cycle in motion – the higher the glucose in the blood, the more insulin is needed to bring it down. We were never designed to eat the volume of sugar we eat today – especially as the body needs the equivalent of only around one teaspoon in the bloodstream at any one time.

Incidentally, you can't just 'burn off' sugar either. We've been under the misapprehension that if we exercise, the offending food will not harm us. It harms every cell – you can't burn off damage. Sugar causes damage to cells in a process called glycation, accelerating the ageing of the body from organs to arteries. It also raises your triglycerides to dangerous levels, which can lead to heart disease.

Too much sugar could result in Type 2 diabetes, caused by insulin resistance. Sugar also promotes infection by slowing the action of white blood cells, which can cause cancer to develop. Sugar is obesogenic, but if you are underweight, sugar is also a very unhealthy way to put weight on, as it presents us with empty calories, no nutrients whatsoever, and ends up actually stripping us of vital nutrients.

In the UK they might contain glucose–fructose syrup, fructose–glucose syrup or isoglucose instead.

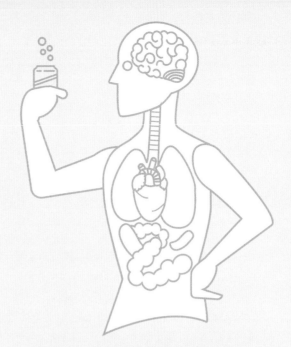

HOW SOFT DRINKS IMPACT YOUR HEALTH

Asthma
Some have reported asthmatic reactions to sodium benzoate, found in soda (fizzy drinks).

Kidney issues
Sodas contain high levels of phosphoric acid, which has been linked to kidney problems.

Sugar overload
After drinking a fizzy drink, you get an insulin burst which turns sugar into fat.

Obesity
For each soda you consume, the risk of obesity increases 1.6 times.

Dissolves tooth enamel
Sugar and acid in soft drinks can dissolve tooth enamel.

Source: Term Life Insurance

Heart disease
Some soft drinks contain high fructose corn syrup which has been associated with an increased risk of metabolic syndrome, associated with heart disease.*

Reproductive issues
Soft drink cans are coated with a resin containing BPA (bisphenol-A), a cancer-causing chemical associated with reproductive abnormalities.

Osteoporosis
Soft drinks contain phosphoric acid which has been associated with bone problems.

Increased risk of diabetes
Those who drink more soda have an 80% risk of developing Type 2 diabetes.

INSULIN.

More sugar means more insulin is released. Insulin has its own set of problems. In excess, it:

- Causes weight gain because it's a fat-promoting hormone.
- Lowers cellular levels of magnesium – this mineral is essential for keeping blood vessels relaxed and maintaining good circulation.
- Increases sodium retention, which in some people may cause hypertension – in others it will result in water retention and discomfort.
- Possibly poses a higher risk for cancer due to insulin's ability to contribute to cell proliferation.
- Increases inflammatory compounds in the blood, damaging the blood vessel walls encouraging excess blood clotting.
- Reduces good HDL cholesterol levels but at the same time the unwelcome smaller LDL cholesterol particles escalate, as do triglycerides, all of which increase the risk for heart disease.

These questions may be helpful in finding out whether you are insulin resistant or not:

Answer YES or NO to the following questions:

- Is getting up in the morning very difficult, especially without coffee?
- Is bread one of your favourite foods? Would you hate to give it up?

- Does exercise leave you exhausted, or are you just too tired to even try?
- Do you shudder at the thought of giving up sugar?
- Do you experience drowsiness after eating?
- Are your moods all over the place?
- Do you struggle to lose weight and find you are putting on even more?
- Would you say you are short of energy most of the time?
- Does going without food for too long make you moody and shaky?
- Would you call yourself an aggressive person when you are hungry?
- Do you get headaches and/or night sweats often?
- Is concentration an issue for you?
- Is alcohol becoming a daily need?
- Do you suffer from hypertension?
- Have you noticed brown/white skin tags around your neck and/or under your arms?
- Have you noticed darkened areas of skin anywhere on your body?
- If you have had blood tests and know your results:
  - Is your LDL high and HDL low?
  - Is your blood sugar too high?
  - Is your insulin level elevated?
  - Is your triglyceride level raised?

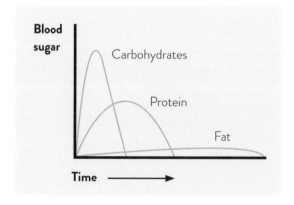

If you answered YES to more than five of the above questions, it is possible that you could be insulin resistant.

FRUCTOSE.

The sugar used for tea and coffee is half fructose and half glucose. Fructose not only causes fatty liver, which leads to diabetes and heart disease, but causes unhealthy weight gain, too. There is an awful lot of bad science and misinformation about fructose, mostly provided by self-taught so-called health experts. Fructose is not a safe sugar alternative – and especially not if you have a fatty liver, diabetes, cancer or heart disease.

In a nutshell, here's what fructose does to the body:

- Promotes obesity
- Causes fatty liver
- Leads to insulin resistance
- It is instrumental in both gout and heart disease
- Is a significant factor in digestive and bowel problems

SUGAR SUBSTITUTES.

There are those who will struggle to give up sugar more than others, and if that's you, well, there is a little ray of hope. Swapping one addiction for another is never a great idea, but there are some safe sweeteners you can use until you muster the courage to let go entirely. In the interim, using erythritol, xylitol or stevia is a safe way to transition to that state of sugar-free living we all need to aspire to.

Erythritol

Erythritol occurs naturally in fruit such as pears, raspberries, melons, grapes, mushrooms and fermented foods and has no carbohydrate or caloric content. Since early 1990s, it has been enjoyed mainly for its closeness in taste to sugar, without the cooling after-taste. It's also superb for baking, but is only approximately 75 per cent as sweet as sugar so more may be needed. Unlike xylitol, it isn't hygroscopic (it doesn't attract moisture), nor does it promote tooth decay the way sugar does. Erythritol has excellent digestive tolerance and is eliminated by the body in under 24 hours with very little absorption. Most of all, it doesn't appear to have any side effects and is very safe.

Erythritol has these properties:

- Calorie-free
- Carb-free
- No digestive issues
- Safe for diabetics (no effect on insulin or blood glucose levels)
- Doesn't cause dental caries
- Completely safe according to the Joint FAO/WHO Expert Committee on Food Additives (JECFA)

Xylitol

The beauty of xylitol is that it has virtually no carbs; it's metabolised as a fibre. It tastes and looks almost identical to sugar, though it has a slight cooling effect on the tongue. Xylitol occurs naturally in the human body, and the enzymes needed to digest it are produced by us as well. It's found in many different varieties of fruit and vegetables. There are many therapeutic benefits, such as prevention of dental caries.

According to endocrinologist Dr Diana Schwarzbein, one of xylitol's benefits includes the ability to stabilise insulin. She points out that a healthy insulin response is essential to healthy ageing and healthy hormones, as well as incidence of hypertension, Type 2 diabetes, and much more. Many toothpastes today contain xylitol as an anti-plaque, anti-bacterial measure. Evidence suggests that it could also be valuable in bone-building and bone health. Dating back to the early 1960s, it's been used widely as a safe and pleasant alternative to sugar.

NB: *Please be aware that xylitol is toxic to animals, especially dogs, but not to humans.*

Stevia

Belonging to the sunflower family, stevia is actually an herb – *Stevia rebaudiana*. Just taste a leaf next time you are at the nursery or buy a bush. It has been around for centuries, originates from Paraguay, and is often called sweet leaf or sugar leaf. It contains no carbs, and is a super alternative to sugar as it has no calories. There are also no side effects whatsoever. It's great for baking, reduces appetite and helps to balance blood sugar. It even has some traces of nutrients present. It is said to soothe heartburn and indigestion – but that seems a bit far-fetched given the small amount one uses. Maybe chewing the leaves would do that more efficiently.

How much sugar do you eat in a day?

Starchy carbs are very high in sugar. To extrapolate how many teaspoons of sugar you are getting from your carbohydrates (the body doesn't know the difference as it essentially converts starch to glucose) – you need to divide your carb grams by four to get the equivalent teaspoons of sugar present.

Let's say a bowl of cereal has 24 grams of carbs (read the labels) then divide that by four to get the equivalent of six teaspoons of sugar. Therefore, carbs divided by four equals the equivalent teaspoons of sugar. All counts following are total carbs, and may give you an idea of how much sugar it's possible to ingest in a day.

BREAKFAST (A high-carb breakfast according to the USDA pyramid) – or 'normal' breakfast

FOOD OR BEVERAGE ITEM	CARBS	SUGAR EQUIVALENT IN TEASPOONS
1 glass boxed 100% fruit juice 250ml	31g	7¾ tsp
25g cornflakes	24.28g	6 tsp
120ml whole milk	6g	1½ tsp
1 teaspoon sugar over the top	4g	1 tsp
1 slice wholewheat bread*	18g	4½ tsp
Butter	0g	0 tsp
1 tablespoon apricot jam	12.88g	3¼ tsp
1 low-fat yoghurt (fruit) 125g	20.8g	5¼ tsp
1 cup coffee, 60ml milk and 1 sugar	7g	1¾ tsp
Potential sugar count:		31 tsp

MID-MORNING (you're hungry now...) tea time/breakfast

1 energy bar – 'healthy' variety, very small	24g	6 tsp
1 small fizzy drink instead of tea	36g	9 tsp
1 slice of bread with egg	18g	4½ tsp
Potential sugar count:		19½ tsp

LUNCH (conservative school lunch)

4 slices wholewheat brown bread*	72g	18 tsp
2 slices regular ham	2.14g	½ tsp
Tomato and butter	0	0
Potential sugar count:		18½ tsp

SUPPER

200g cooked spaghetti	42.95g (43g)	10¾ tsp
Bolognaise*	4g	1 tsp
Bread roll, white	26g	6½ tsp
Red wine, one glass	3.84g (4g)	1 tsp
Potential sugar count:		19¼ tsp

Potential total for the day excluding TV nibbles and afternoon tea:	88¼ tsp

This is what is *possible*. Imagine now adding in more alcohol, coffees throughout the day, more wine and between-meal snacks – and a pudding? The mind boggles.

Values for bread, bolognaise and spaghetti are from fatsecret.co.za. Bread values based on Low GI Sasko wholewheat brown loaf at 18 carbs per slice, although some brands are higher in other databases.

On the other hand, here's what a sensible low-carb day could look like:

BREAKFAST

FOOD OR BEVERAGE ITEM	CARBS	SUGAR CONTENT
2 large eggs in butter	0.3g	
3 rashers of bacon	0.2g	
Wilted spinach, 1 cup (180g)	1.09g	
½ avocado (small 50g incl shell)	4.5g	Not quite 2 tsp sugar equivalent and you won't be hungry for hours!
40g cherry tomatoes	1g	
Coffee, no sugar, with 1 tbsp cream	0.4g	
Total	7.49g	

LUNCH (if you need it – you won't need morning snacks for sure!)

Big salad with 75g lettuce leaves shredded	1.63g	
80g tomatoes	1g	
50g cucumber slices	1.89g	
225g tinned tuna (1 tin)	0g	
Olive oil 1-2 tbsp	0g	Just over 1 tsp of sugar
Apple cider vinegar 1 tbsp	0g	
Rooibos tea/coffee/leaf tea with no milk or sugar	0.4g	
Total	4.92g	

SUPPER

Piece of steak 100-200g	0g	
165g cauliflower (cooked)	3g	
90g broccoli (cooked)	3.4g	2½ tsp sugar
75g cabbage ribbons in butter	2.4g	
Cream sauce with sour cream	1.2g	
Total	10g	

The entire day (excluding extras) could in fact come to the equivalent of **5-6 tsp sugar**.

ARTIFICIAL SWEETENERS.

Acesulfame K

This is a sweetener found in protein shakes and beverages, which contains methylene chloride – a known carcinogen. Long-term exposure to methylene chloride found in Acesulfame K causes nausea, headaches, mood problems, impairment of the liver and kidneys, problems with eyesight and cancer. Lab tests conducted on rats showed multiple cancer developments including leukaemia and chronic respiratory disease. It also stimulates insulin secretion and can worsen reactive hypoglycaemia. To make matters worse, it is often found paired with aspartame.

Aspartame

There are over 90 documented symptoms listed in reports on the consumption of aspartame, a chemical poison that can cause seizures, chronic fatigue, panic attacks, anxiety and depression, but there are many more sinister illnesses as well.

Cyclamates and saccharin

Cyclamates were banned by the US Food and Drug Administration (FDA) for consumption by humans in 1969, but are currently still being used in at least 45 other countries. The UK government advises restricting intake of cyclamate in children. Cyclamates are 30 to 50 times sweeter than sugar but it's the least sweet of all artificial sweeteners, often combined with saccharin in a 1:10 ratio to improve its taste. Cyclamates do not occur in nature and early studies in the 1970s linked the combination of saccharin and cyclamates to increased bladder cancer in lab animals.

Sucralose

Sucralose, or Splenda, is not the harmless alternative to sugar it's made out to be. Dr Ralph Hyman states categorically that it causes obesity. Hang on, isn't this supposed to prevent obesity? Many people mistakenly feel they are preventing weight gain by popping some artificial chemical into their tea or coffee, when in fact they are increasing their chances of weight gain.

The US consumer watchdog group, the Center for Science in the Public Interest (CSPI), has recently downgraded sucralose from a 'safe' to a 'caution' rating after there was a leukaemia scare. Dr Joseph Mercola explains: "It's a chlorinated artificial sweetener in line with aspartame and saccharin, with detrimental health effects to match."

Chapter

02

WHY WE SHOULD AVOID GRAINS

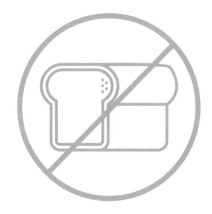

We avoid grains in any shape or form on LCHF as they are inherently bad for the body, and may cause numerous digestive problems. Gluten is one of the key problem areas in grains like wheat, rye, barley and spelt. Some would argue oats do not contain gluten, but they are generally contaminated with it since they are produced in facilities where other gluten-containing grains are processed. Oats are still a high-carb grain, gluten or not.

Gluten is the generic term used for a mixture of proteins found in all grains, and different grains even contain different types of gluten. The wheat we have today is not the wheat of the Bible and, despite what you may believe, that kind of wheat actually doesn't exist anymore. In the last 30 to 50 years, there have been more changes made to our food than in the last several thousand years. Today's wheat has been manipulated to contain 50 per cent more gluten than 50 years ago; it's hybridised, interfered with and has become something completely unnatural.

Our aversion to grains is not only about gluten but while we are on the subject, gluten is made up of sub-fractions (small pieces of protein) called prolamins and glutelins, and wheat is typically the most detrimental of all grains as it contains the prolamine called gliadin, to which many people react severely. Some of the gluten prolamine proteins found in grains and the percentage of total protein that is prolamine include:

Wheat	69% gliadin
Barley	46-52% hordein
Rye	30-50% secalinin
Oats	16% avenin
Corn	55% zein
Millet	40% pacenin
Rice	5% orzenin

You'll be forgiven if you have never heard of any of these before. However, if you are suffering constantly from any of the following conditions listed below, it could be that even though you are not aware of it, or tests have proved negative for gluten intolerance (remember gluten is only one of the proteins in grain), you are still suffering the effects of one or more of these proteins on your body:

- Fatigue
- Joint pain
- Inflammation
- Balance problems, dizziness
- Numbness, tingling
- Depression, irritability
- Mood swings
- Anxiety
- Brain fog
- Headaches/migraines
- Skin rashes
- Keratosis pilaris (chicken skin on arms)
- Anaemia
- Hormone imbalances
- Respiratory problems
- Digestive problems, even though you are eating a traditional gluten-free diet

Gluten interferes with zonulin, which keeps the cells that line our digestive tract stuck together, by so-called 'tight junctions', preventing any proteins and waste products from entering the bloodstream. Gluten stimulates zonulin and is responsible for causing a condition called 'leaky gut', where the gut lining becomes permeable, resulting in a laundry list of symptoms such as allergies, autoimmune diseases and asthma.

It's an irritant to the bowel and a very common cause of bowel inflammation, from irritable bowel syndrome and Crohn's disease to ulcerative colitis and more.

The bowel wall is lined with tiny finger-like projections called villi to increase its surface area, and they are responsible for the absorption of all the nutrients from your food. Inflammation in the bowel can cause the breakdown of these villi which means that your ability to absorb nutrients diminishes dramatically and you are short-changed on your nutrition.

Bread and gluten are notorious for causing digestive disturbances such as bloating, gas and constipation. The majority of people notice a significant, almost immediate difference in the way they feel by simply reducing or eliminating grains from their diet. Constipation diminishes, gas and bloating disappears and nutrient absorption increases, including iron levels. If you are anaemic, gluten may just be the culprit, as it decreases iron uptake.

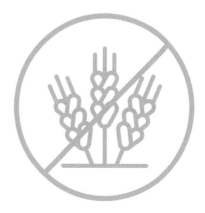

Wheat contains an appetite stimulant derived from the digestion of the gliadin protein which yields exorphins or exogenous morphine-like compounds. Bread can be just as addictive as sugar. Most supermarket bread contains much more gluten than would occur in nature, as it is made from modified short grain wheat which contains more gluten than the original grains – plus large amounts of extra gluten are added to bread to extend shelf life. Commercial breads are also very poorly fermented, having been whipped up and baked on a production line within an hour or two. Proper fermentation should take eight hours or more.

Decades ago, instead of yeast, bakers would use a starter culture which takes a few days to prepare and ripen. Proper fermentation helps to break down gluten and other compounds in the bread, making it much easier to digest. Of course, whether you use this kind of bread of not, it's all high-carb – so forget it, just dump the grains.

Gliadorphins are incompletely broken down 'pieces of gluten' which react with opiate receptors in the brain; this mimics the effects of opiate drugs like heroin and morphine, thus giving gluten an almost addictive effect. Like opiate drugs, when gluten binds to your brain's opiate receptors, you can experience momentary positive effects like mood elevation, confidence and calm, even an emotional attachment to bread verging on the addictive. Long-term consumption may cause regular mood swings, bowel disturbances, weight gain, reflux, anxiety or depression.

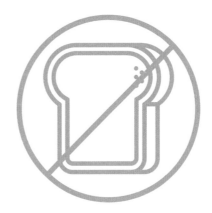

Gluten also dramatically affects your blood sugar balance. Eating bread is just like eating sugar – it even has a higher glycaemic index than sugar. All flour is a type of starch which is made up of a chain of sugars. When you digest starch, it is broken down into glucose by the body. This causes a blood-sugar spike, giving you a satisfying energy high, followed by an energy slump shortly afterwards, and leaves you craving more starchy or sugary food, and so the cycle continues. Break your dependence, and many of your mystery complaints will disappear.

Gluten's a problem, no doubt about it – it makes you put on weight. But that's not entirely the reason we avoid wheat – there's more to it than that. It's a contributor to heart disease, obesity, thyroid dysfunction, cancer, dementia, depression and many other distressing illnesses. Even in those who eat a lot of wheat due to poverty – they are malnourished – it is a nutrient robber and is nutrient-poor. Sadly, wheat is in so many other products, too – from sauces to medications and almost every foodstuff you purchase that is not a single-ingredient food item. The wheat of today is not the wheat our great grandmothers used; and even then, nobody ate a fraction of the bread and grain products people eat today.

'SUPER' WHEAT.

Modern wheat contains a 'super' starch called Amylopectin A, which is super fattening. It also contains a form of super gluten, which is super inflammatory. The bread we consume these days is like a super drug, making it highly addictive to the point of people saying they just cannot do without bread.

In his book *Wheat Belly*, Dr William Davis tells the story of wheat – how it has changed dramatically from the Einkorn wheat of Bible days, to the horrific monster we know as wheat today. It does untold damage to our bodies, it's literally a 'Frankenwheat'. Modern wheat is dwarf wheat, hybridised beyond recognition and genetically manipulated to produce higher yields, more gluten, and more starch. In fact, the man who engineered modern wheat won a Nobel Prize, it was so changed from how nature presents it to us.

Amylopectin A is the reason wheat is so wonderfully fluffy when baked. Yet, what this also does is raise your blood sugar disproportionately. It is scary to think a slice of bread will raise your blood sugar more than a tablespoon of sugar. And there is no difference between white and wholewheat, by the way – bread is bread – and the wholegrain story is a creative one to make you think you are eating more healthily. Both raise blood sugar to the same extent.

Avoid wheat and grains if you want good health and longevity. Your daily bread will give you a bread belly (or a "wheat belly", as Davis puts it), trigger enormous inflammation in the body and may provide you with a fatty liver as a bonus. This causes a cascade of disease from obesity to diabetes to cardiovascular disease. It's just not worth it.

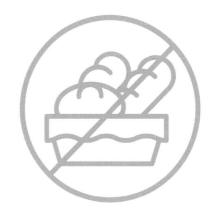

Chapter

02

THE PROBLEM WITH SOYA AND CORN

SOYA.

There is the misguided notion that soya is a viable alternative to animal protein, and vegetarians mistakenly believe it to be a healthy substitute for meat, which it is not for many reasons. It also causes weight gain.

Plant protein and animal protein are poles apart. Suffice it to say, soya is a harmful non-food, and as a legume (the worst of them), it's fraught with problems from the protease inhibitors and saponins to phytates and lectins.

But apart from that, it is not good for you for many reasons. Here are just a few:

- *There are hormone disruptors present in soya, and these in particular interfere with thyroid function – from slowing it down, to causing auto-immune thyroid conditions, even cancer.*

- *Soya has rather nasty trypsin inhibitors (an important enzyme) which therefore interferes with protein digestion and muscle growth.*

- *Soya is very high in phytates and lectins, which block the body's ability to absorb important minerals like calcium, magnesium, zinc and copper. Processed soya also leads to an increased risk of fatty liver disease while significantly blocking the uptake of iron, leading to iron-deficiency anaemia.*

- *Virtually all the soya on the planet is genetically modified. That makes it off limits for low-carbers – and not a real food. It has to undergo a lot of processing just to make it edible.*

- *Soya lacks two very important essential amino acids: methionine and cysteine. Therefore it is not a 'complete' protein – only animal flesh is a complete protein, as it has all 22 amino acids present.*

- *Soya creates an increased need for Vitamin D in the diet.*

- *The B12 present is an analogue, and actually causes B12 deficiency.*

- *Unlike animal protein, there is no Vitamin A present in soya. There is a mistaken notion that there is sufficient Vitamin A in the form of beta-carotene; however, this is very poorly converted into Vitamin A, if at all. Without sufficient Vitamin A in the diet, we lay ourselves open to infection, poor bone density, eye and reproductive disorders.*
- *Most soya will have MSG (monosodium glutamate) added to it, to make it taste a bit better. MSG is a neurotoxic taste enhancer.*

There is much to be said about soya – an excellent read is *The Whole Soy Story* by Dr Kaayla Daniel. All you need do is Google "soya dangers" for more information.

CORN.

Corn is now one of the biggest crops in the world for feeding livestock and human beings (especially in the USA), *but corn is not a vegetable*, it's a grain or seed-head of grass. South Africa's indigenous people rely heavily on corn – it is regarded as a staple food. From corn comes corn syrup, high fructose corn syrup, polenta, maize starch, corn starch, maltodextrin and various other corn products. Most of it,

unbelievably, is consumed by animals globally – livestock are given corn as a staple food to fatten them – a food they were never meant to eat. Corn makes both animals and people sick and overweight. It's high in inflammatory omega-6 fats, displacing beneficial omega-3 when eaten regularly. Forget the corn if you want to live LCHF, it's just another grain – corn is not a vegetable.

Whether you are eating baby corn or sweetcorn, you are eating a grain. Remember, corn in any disguise is almost always genetically modified, although there are some nutritional benefits if organic. The LCHF paradigm does not include grains in any shape or form.

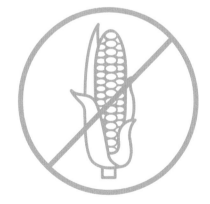

Chapter

02

THE DAIRY DEBATE

The dairy debate is probably one of the hottest topics in the LCHF world today. Some streams include it while others condemn it, but by far the most common problem appears to be 'dairy overdosing'. We simply eat too many dairy products. It's really not as healthy as it's made out to be, and is best avoided for most people, although some tolerate dairy better than others.

In a perfect world, raw organic dairy from pasture-fed cows would be first prize – along the lines of the Dr Weston A Price philosophy. However, there are still inherent problems. Raw, pasture-fed products free from antibiotics, growth promoters, steroids and grain feed are thin on the ground and are even outlawed in some countries. Perhaps a good approach to dairy would be as an occasional indulgence, much the way alcohol, chocolate and cake (LCHF, of course) should be enjoyed. Daily consumption of grass-fed butter is encouraged as this is the fat, without the milk proteins.

THE PALEO VIEW.

Paleo is the largest and fastest-growing low-carb movement on the planet today, so it's something which needs to be covered. Paleo for the most part steers clear of dairy entirely. Professor Loren Cordain, one of the leaders of the Paleo movement, is anti-dairy and has some very good points on why it should not be included in a healthy diet.

Some of the points he cites in his book, *The Paleo Answer*, include the following:

- Compared to meat, fruit and vegetables, dairy lacks nutritional density.
- Milk is an incredibly insulinogenic food – causing disproportionate blood insulin spiking to take place.
- Hormones present in milk and dairy products affect our hormones; one such hormone, insulin-like growth factor (IGF-1), has been associated strongly with breast and prostate cancer.
- Leaky gut may be a result of regular dairy consumption due to protease inhibitors.
- Dairy is a powerful factor in all respiratory illness as it increases mucus production. Asthmatics, sinus sufferers and atopic people would all be well advised to avoid dairy. It not only affects the respiratory tract, but does the same in the gastrointestinal tract by irritating the gut lining.
- Dairy is one of the most allergenic of all foods, and many people who embark on a LCHF diet do so not only for weight loss, but for improved health. Dairy intolerance is alarmingly common, and may actively prevent weight loss.

THE LCHF VIEW.

At the other end of the spectrum, dairy fat (butter, ghee) and fermented dairy can be very beneficial for some people, with the proviso being that it is sourced from pasture-fed cows only, as it's a good source of fat-soluble vitamins, conjugated linoleic acid and probiotics.

When we wrote the red book, we decided we wanted to include dairy products, as we chose the Scandinavian stream of LCHF, where dairy features heavily. The problem here is that we are in South Africa, and the Scandinavians are the only people, except for a few European countries like Netherlands, who tolerate dairy products exceptionally well. We are not as fortunate, but we included it anyway, and it has become a pillar of LCHF in this country. That doesn't mean it is right or good in every case. Nobody has all the truth and the understanding of LCHF is still in its infancy. We need to keep an open mind, and not allow our intelligence to degenerate to that of believing any one group of people mindlessly without further investigation. The most-learned people have been wrong before – and dairy certainly presents many challenges to most LCHF followers.

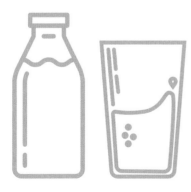

CHILDREN.

It is argued that dairy could be beneficial for children. However, there are two very distinct schools of thought here. One stream says no mammal would drink the milk of another mammal after weaning; whereas others would say children need the nutrients and minerals in milk for bones, teeth and growth. Provided that it's not introduced too early, dairy can be tolerated by most children. There are all sorts of arguments about how long to breastfeed and whether this makes a difference. We won't get into that here, but in some ways, the science is still unclear. Butter though, is always encouraged unless there is clear intolerance to it.

The proteins in milk are very strong cross-reactive foods with gluten, so those with gluten-intolerance or coeliac disease are advised to avoid dairy products, and this applies to all forms of dairy, even butter in some instances. People can be intolerant to either the lactose (sugar) or the casein (protein) fraction of milk and either could cause weight gain or failure to lose weight, skin and respiratory problems, digestive distress or mood disorders. As youngsters, we usually have a lot more of the enzyme lactase to digest milk; yet as we age and our immune systems deteriorate, stress manifests and we are not as

67

resilient as we were when younger. We are less able to digest lactose and all our enzymes, lactase included, diminish.

TOO MUCH OF A GOOD THING.

If dairy products were eaten sparingly or infrequently, we'd probably see far fewer problems. For example, in a person who has five cups of tea or coffee with milk a day, daily yoghurt for breakfast, cheese at lunch and a milk or cheese sauce at dinner – one can expect more problems than the person who largely avoids it and has the odd piece of cheese once a week. It may well be the sheer volume of dairy we eat today coupled with the hormones, homogenisation and pasteurisation that causes the problem. They are all contributing factors.

If you have an auto-immune disease, asthma, arthritis or any inflammatory problem, you might want to try a month or two without dairy, and then reintroduce it and see what happens. This is why dairy is such a truly grey area.

Butter is pretty self-limiting, so it's unlikely anyone would overeat it, but cheese, yoghurt, milk and cream are easy to overdo. While goat's products are kinder to the body, in many they present the same challenges as dairy.

Dairy does tend to make cooking and living in general, easier, but are we after an easy life or a healthy life? If dairy triggers allergies or

inflammation, it may not be worth the trouble. It's pretty addictive, too. You need time to adjust if you choose to stop dairy and you also need to find alternatives.

Regarding weight loss, dairy appears to inhibit it, *particularly* in women. About 15 per cent of women seem fine on dairy, but for the most part there comes that time when they plateau and cannot lose any more weight – that's probably the best time to ditch the dairy. Even some men find this. So if your scales are 'stuck', try dropping dairy, you may be pleasantly surprised. Women have a love affair with dairy and can seldom have just a little dairy: it's an all-or-nothing relationship.

Dairy products, particularly milk and yoghurt, are extremely insulinogenic (elevate insulin levels); sticking with butter and a little hard cheese may still be okay for some. Cows have over 80 other naturally occurring hormones which are not 'human' and which affect our hormones.

This begs the question: should we be having any at all? Butter is generally free from these hormones as the hormones are in the protein fraction of the milk, but if you are particularly sensitive, this may

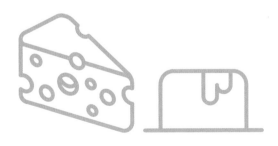

have more of an effect on you than you realise. Certain people can tolerate a little occasionally, while others need to cut it out completely to see results.

CALCIUM.

But where to get one's calcium is a common refrain. The simple answer is that we have an enormous amount of beautiful, bioavailable calcium in our food. The Vitamins D and K2 from egg yolks, fish, pasture-fed butter and grass-fed beef all help to increase uptake of calcium, which is actually quite prevalent in the diet. Preferably, do not take calcium supplements. There is too much evidence that it lands up in the wrong places like the arteries, soft tissues and brain, not the bones.

Remember, there are plenty of dairy-free calcium-rich foods, including:

- *All dark, leafy greens*
- *Almond milk*
- *Bok choy*
- *Carrots*
- *Chicken livers*
- *Homemade bone broth*
- *Oysters and seafood*
- *Sardines and tinned fish in brine with bones crushed into the fish*
- *Sesame seeds*
- *Nuts*

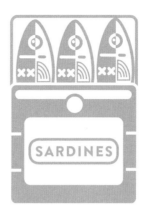

We only need around 300 to 400 milligrams of calcium daily, so by eating some of the above foods daily – particularly leafy greens with bioavailable calcium – you will get enough. You may get too much calcium from supplements which could cause kidney stones but dietary calcium is generally safe. Breakfast cereals, crackers and various foods are usually fortified with too much calcium, another reason to avoid processed foods. Greens are packed with magnesium too – calcium is not properly assimilated without magnesium, and nature presents it to us in a perfect package. Vitamins K2 and D3 make dietary calcium safe, and deliver it straight to the bones, literally "keeping calcium in its place".

An overlooked reason to eat probiotic-rich foods (including sauerkraut, kimchi and kefir) is to increase healthy bacteria. These, in turn, will help to absorb more dietary calcium. Coconut milk and homemade almond milk are excellent dairy alternatives.

03

MYTHS AND MISCONCEPTIONS

Myths are a waste of time. They prevent progression.

– Barbara Streisand

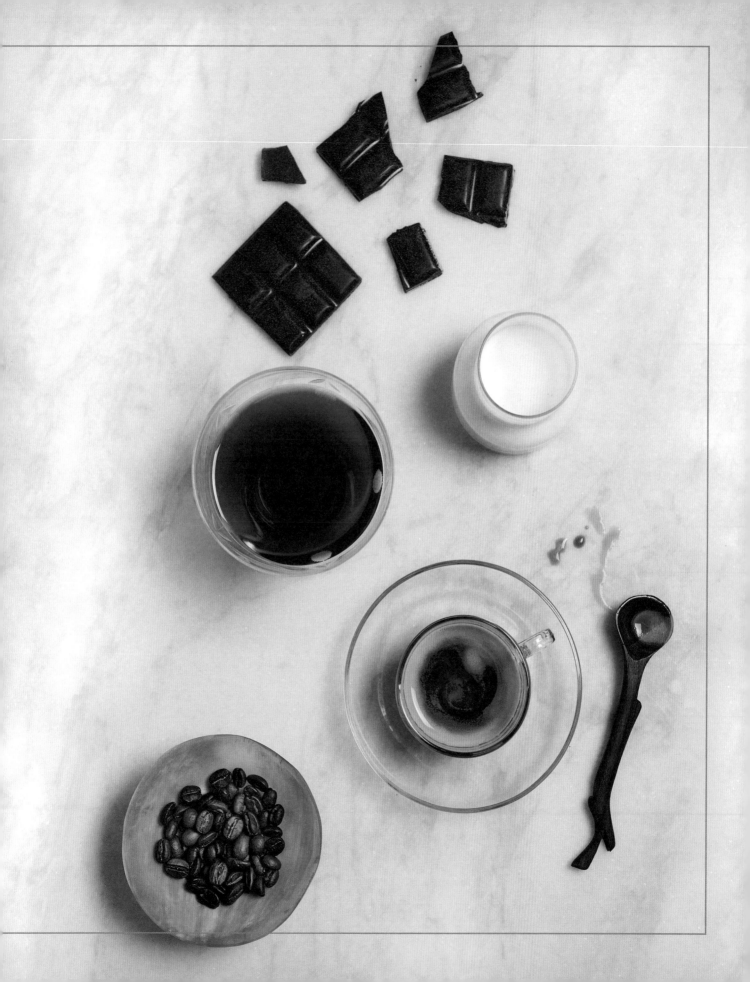

Chapter

03

DIETARY DECEPTIONS

Nutritional and dietary advice is classically fraught with wrong information. Here are a few myths which need to be laid to rest, now and forever.

SATURATED FAT IS DANGEROUS FOR YOUR HEART.

This is a terrible misrepresentation of the truth. Saturated fat is crucial in protecting our nerves, for the manufacture of hormones and maintenance of cell membranes. Saturated fats enable the body to absorb the all-important fat-soluble Vitamins A, D, E and K, which support mucous membrane health, bone and tooth health, antioxidant status and efficient blood clotting, just to name a few of their functions. The human body needs animal fats in the diet – the old low-fat, fat-free diets are extremely unhealthy and do absolutely nothing but make us ill. Contrary to popular opinion, animal fat is extremely nutritious. Sources of animal fat such as eggs, butter, meat, lard, suet, full-fat milk and cheese are all healthy. Coconut oil is also a good saturated fat.

In the 1970s we were told some porkies:

- *Fat – especially saturated fat – is the enemy, and it is still called "artery-clogging saturated fat" as though this was all one word.*
- *Fat will raise cholesterol which will cause heart disease.*
- *If you develop high cholesterol, you will need statin drugs.*
- *Instead of fat, use vegetable oils (seed oils) and margarine; light, low-fat, fat-free and non-saturated fat alternatives – cut fat right down or out.*
- *Fat makes you fat.*

All of the above are untrue. Fat is healthy, good, wonderful, tasty, satisfying and to be enjoyed. However, just because fat has no carbohydrate value, don't overdo it; enjoy it sensibly.

VEGETABLE OIL FALLACY.

Vegetable fats and oils are extremely harmful to health; they cause inflammation and disease, and really don't taste good either. Such oils include soya, cottonseed, safflower, sunflower, grapeseed, canola, corn, flaxseed, margarine and oil blends. Never buy anything with these oils in again if you value your health. They are all seed or grain oils.

MARGARINE VERSUS BUTTER.

I think we all know by now that margarine is the chemical, plastic equivalent of butter. It's tragic that people believe that this man-made goo should be viewed as a healthy food; how far we have fallen. Butter is a natural, wholefood packed with nutrition and the hard-to-find valuable Vitamin K2 – which is completely lacking in margarine. Don't be deceived, margarine is a damaged, dangerous, highly inflammatory, highly processed non-food. Butter is real food.

THE LOW-FAT LIE.

This really is a serious lie – and the past 50 years have taught us that this doesn't work. Fat does not make you fat, but eating a low-fat diet does seem to have a devastating influence on our health, obesity, heart disease and diabetes. Low-fat comes with low taste, and therefore artificial sweeteners or sugar must be added to supply flavour, so low-fat products are by default virtually always high-carb.

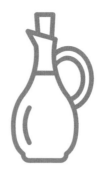

CHOLESTEROL WILL CLOG YOUR ARTERIES.

Doesn't everyone know by now that this was based on bad science and is *totally* wrong? The truth has been greatly stretched, according to mountains of scientific literature. Cholesterol is crucial to good health. It acts as a very powerful antioxidant, it's needed by your liver to make bile, and it helps prevent depression. Cholesterol repairs tears in your arteries and blood vessels, is vital for your brain and nervous system to function properly and helps your body manufacture Vitamin D. All your sex hormones are made from cholesterol.

The real culprit behind clogged arteries is chronic inflammation, which appears to be a direct result of a low-fat, high-carbohydrate diet rich in omega-6 fatty acids, found mostly in harmful seed oils and processed food. The cholesterol found in arterial plaque is a protective response to the damage caused by inflammation; blaming cholesterol is like blaming firefighters for causing a fire.

ALL CALORIES ARE CREATED EQUAL.

Anyone knows that calories from cabbage and calories from sweets will have completely different effects on the body. Remember, food is information and good information provides fuel and nutrition to the body – bad information in the form of sugar and junk food will make you tired, sick and lethargic. You can't just eat X-amount of calories a day no matter where they come from (like fizzy drinks and cakes) – you'd have to be almost brain-dead to believe these can be any good for you. It's all about nourishing food, not just a caloric number.

A LITTLE SUGAR'S FINE.

No, sorry, this is false. No amount of sugar is safe. Cane sugar, or sucrose, is 50 per cent glucose and 50 per cent fructose. Fructose and glucose are very different, and are metabolised differently. Every cell uses glucose and it's burned for energy. Fructose is stored as fat. If you want to be fat, eat fructose.

You will also place strain on your liver by eating too much fructose because it creates waste products like uric acid, which raises your blood pressure, is responsible for gout, and causes both fatty liver disease and heart disease – and that's just for starters, as half the sugar molecule is fructose, so even a little is not okay.

WHOLEGRAINS ARE PART OF A HEALTHY DIET.

This is a whopper! All women know that they will get fat on grains, whether they are wholegrains, refined grains or cereal grains. There is simply no such thing as a healthy wholegrain, nor a healthy grain, period. Grains are extremely unhealthy for the human body in the long term. Experts like Dr William Davis have an awful lot to say about the damage wheat and some other grains do to the entire body, starting in the digestive tract.

Why are some slim people prone to heart attacks and other dread diseases? We are all unique genetically, and while some people may not gain weight from a grain-based diet, they are still prone to the damage grains cause to the gut. Therefore, while some grain-eaters may not gain weight, their arteries and brains are still affected by grain's inflammatory nature.

DAIRY IS ESSENTIAL TO LCHF.

Wrong again. A large number of LCHF followers have had to forego dairy to continue their weight loss journey and healthy lifestyle. More and more people simply do not tolerate dairy – and most certainly not in the vast amounts that people consume it. Unfortunately, dairy being a relatively 'free' food in the red book, led to people going overboard with it and having way too much. Too much of anything is never a good thing; too much water and your brain will swell and you will die. We need to use common sense. This is part of the reason for creating a Gold list and placing dairy on that list. You will see it also appears in grey areas and on the Grey list later on. Paleo followers completely avoid dairy.

ALL-DAY GRAZING KEEPS BLOOD SUGAR STABLE.

Where this came from is a mystery. By continually eating or eating six small meals a day, you constantly keep blood sugar and insulin levels raised, and weight loss will be difficult. Blood sugar isn't at all stable (unless you call high blood sugar all day 'stable') and it's really unhealthy anyway. Give your body a chance to digest its last meal and you'll get better results.

Continual hunger will be a thing of the past if you eat a low-carb diet, as you won't need to nibble all day. People who live on sugar and carbs do get hungry often, as they have endless blood sugar highs and lows requiring more food. In fact, going to the other extreme of intermittent fasting (eating once or twice a day) is much healthier for you. But just eating three solid meals a day is a good start.

'FOOD COMBINING' IS HEALTHY.

The theory here is that you should never eat protein and carbs together – but all food other than animal protein and fat comes packaged with carbs, fat and protein. Our digestive enzymes and magnificent bodies are well able to handle anything in any mixture – that's how we were created. Forget the fads, there are dozens of them, this is just another useless one. Stick with proper physiology and solid science.

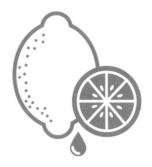

THE PH ACID/ALKALINE MYTH.

Despite what you have been told, no food can change the pH of the body. There is not an ounce of credible, scientific evidence whatsoever to back this up. Your stomach has hydrochloric acid almost as strong as battery acid to help the enzyme pepsin to break proteins into peptones. That is how you were created, and to think you can interfere is to not understand how the body works at all. Different parts of your body have a different pH; which one are you wanting to alkalanize? Is it saliva, stomach acid, skin, duodenum, small intestine, bladder, large intestine, urine or blood? They all have different levels of acidity – or pH levels. A shift in blood pH by a minuscule amount can be fatal, so it's clearly not the blood.

The truth is nothing can or should get past your stomach acid; it is too powerful and that is exactly how it is meant to be. Urine can be affected, but this is not an accurate predictor of the body's acidity whatsoever – the kidneys tightly regulate the body's pH, and to some degree the lungs do, too. All the nonsense about acid and alkaline is really another fad that has no place in science.

CHILDREN NEED FRUIT JUICE.

There is the misconception that fruit juice is safer and healthier than fizzy drinks, and that children need juice. Not so fast. This is just another way to ingest excess sugar and have the kids bouncing off the wall.

Think about the commercial juices you buy. They all have the same syrupy consistency, but a vaguely different flavour. Juice is not syrupy in nature, it is watery. Read the side of the pack or bottle and check the amount of sugar it contains, but make sure you are sitting down first – it can have from nine to 14 teaspoons of sugar per serving; in fact as much, and sometimes more, than fizzy drinks. Rather give a child fresh fruit instead of juice. Children also need to be taught the value of drinking water. They don't need fruit juice.

SOYA REPLACES MEAT AS A PROTEIN SOURCE.

The thinking in uneducated circles is that soya can take the place of meat and animal protein: well, sorry, it can't. It is a damaging, harmful processed food with nothing going for it.

Why would you want to eat highly processed food instead of real food? Soya is full of xenoestrogens (oestrogen mimics) which wreak havoc on our hormones at every age, may cause cancer and over 90 per cent of the world's soya is genetically modified anyway. This is an endocrine disrupter and can lead to many problems, not least of which is weight gain.

Soya is one of those nasty ubiquitous substances which has crept into almost all processed food and sauces. Just another reason to eat single-ingredient foods that you prepare from scratch.

I ONLY NEED TO AVOID GLUTEN IF I'M COELIAC.

Gluten is toxic to every single one of us, albeit to different degrees. Coeliac disease is an auto-immune condition; however, it doesn't mean if you are not coeliac that you can be gung-ho with the grains. Gluten can be a risk for thyroid cancer in some people, and has a list as long as a person's leg of the problems associated with it, especially when it comes to digestive issues. Always avoid gluten, especially if you have bowel, joint or respiratory problems. As a LCHF eater, you won't be eating grain anyway.

For those of you who think it is okay to have a bowl of pasta or some sort of carbohydrate indulgence once a week, here is a quote Dr Davis, author of *Wheat Belly*, posted on Facebook a while back: "It amazes me that people often mistake weight loss for health – yes, they are related, but not 100 per cent.

Take small LDL particles, for instance, the most common abnormality in people with heart attacks. One indulgence in carbs per week provokes small LDL particles that persist for about seven days. In other words, a once-per-week carb indulgence generates cardiovascular risk for 52 weeks per year." A sobering thought.

RESISTANT STARCH.

The idea that resistant starch (RS) is something good comes from the fact that it is not digested by the body, but by the healthy gut bacteria. This starch is resistant to digestion so passes through the body undigested, similar to fibre, which is incredibly important and essential to health.

There are various forms of RS; some are presented as a man-made chemical process (we don't recommend processed products as they are not real food); another type is found in cooked and chilled potatoes, rice and green-tipped bananas. This is not to say you should hurl yourself headlong into a giant potato salad every day, but now and then including a chilled potato or a green banana appears to be healthy for your gut.

Everything starts and ends with gut health. RS is food for your healthy strains of bacteria and provides an increase in short-chain fatty acids such as butyrate, the preferred fuel of the cells lining the colon, which lowers inflammation. Even in very small amounts, it has been shown to reduce insulin sensitivity and improve metabolism. For some people, it appears to accelerate weight loss. Do your own experimenting.

GMO FOODS ARE HARMLESS.

When scientists displace nature by cutting bits of a living organism's DNA and splicing it into a completely unrelated species, we call this a genetically modified organism (GMO), and it is the furthest thing from natural you can imagine.

There has not been nearly enough time to see what the long-term effects of GMOs are, although some tests that have been carried out have had bad enough results to call GMO food 'Frankenfood'. Genes are incredibly complex, and by altering the genetic code of living organisms, engineers are manipulating the very process of life itself.

But it gets worse; genetic engineers aren't just splicing plant to plant anymore:

- Chicken genes have been introduced into potatoes.
- Fish genes are introduced into strawberries.
- Bacteria and viruses have been introduced into cucumbers and tomatoes.
- Mouse genes have been introduced into tobacco.
- Plus, they're splicing deadly chemical pesticides, herbicides and fungicides directly into the plants themselves now – what on earth are they thinking?

GMO foods are largely untested and humans are the guinea pigs. Jeffrey Smith, author of the book *Seeds of Deception*, has done decades of research on this, and GMOs definitely affect our health adversely. See Smith's website or watch his YouTube clips for some interesting information (see Bibliography page 249).

Doesn't it just feel wrong to think that you are eating a strawberry which is part fish? How do vegans feel about this?

DON'T WE NEED CARBS?

Amazingly, the human being has no fundamental need for carbohydrates – protein is essential and we need essential fats, but there are no essential carbs or sugars. However, anything that is not pure fat or protein does have carbs, and eating them in vegetables is absolutely fine.

Nobody needs bread, sugar, pasta or potatoes, let's be honest. The body can also produce glucose through the process of gluconeogenesis – where glucose (carbs) is made from amino acids and fat by the liver.

WHAT ABOUT FIBRE?

The body needs fibre, definitely. It is vitally important for good bowel health, but it should not come from brans and grains, we should get enough from our plant foods. In a day, the recommendation is around 30 grams of fibre – the question is: can we meet this on a LCHF diet? Absolutely. Remember the carb grams in fibre do not get digested by you, as they are food for the healthy bacteria, and then they are eliminated from the body. You could use psyllium husks if you have irregular bowel habits – one tablespoon has zero grams net carbs, but 10 grams fibre.

WHAT ABOUT FAT FASTS AND FAT BOMBS?

Fat bombs and fat fasts might be fine for men and thin extreme athletes, but life's not fair, and women just don't have that kind of metabolism; neither do most ordinary men. Women appear to metabolise fats very differently to men, so while they must not go on a low-fat diet by any means, they should not embark on a fat fest (forget the fat bombs if you are not a female athlete). They serve no real purpose.

Simply eat the fat on meat, enjoy avocados, a few nuts and seeds, cook with delicious animal fats, put delectable homemade salad dressing on salads, but don't force-feed yourself fat or anything else for that matter – it's totally unnecessary and unnatural. We all eat too much food anyway – getting used to going without food for longer periods is a great way to teach the body to burn fat. The correct proportion of fat to protein needed by a human being is one-quarter fat to three-quarters lean meat. This is more or less what you would find on a fatty, succulent lamb chop.

WHAT ABOUT SPIKING, KETOSIS, INTERMITTENT FASTING, AND OTHER QUICK FIX METHODS?

There's a time and a place for everything, but we don't believe in the spiking theory at all, and we don't need to constantly be in ketosis either. Ketosis is great for diabetics; but, for the ordinary person, there are pros and cons to being in ketosis. For some, there is the possibility of a slower metabolism with time. Intermittent fasting is fine – you can skip a meal or two if you feel okay. Eating two to three well-planned meals a day is still a good idea.

COUNTING CARBS, POINTS, RATIOS.

Eating LCHF has become riddled with rules; it ought not to be so. It should be about eating real food that is lower in carbs, avoiding junk foods, high-carb starchy and sugary foods. Low-carb for one person may be 100 grams a day; for another person it may be 50 grams. It's an individual thing. If you are careful and are losing weight steadily it is not necessary to count carbs obsessively. The best way to do LCHF is to get a feel for how much to eat, which foods are best, and when to eat them. No counting, no panic. But at some point, one of the snags in weight loss will be the dreaded plateau, and it may be that you are simply consuming too many carbs without realising it. This is where you may want to keep track of your carb consumption. See the new updated lists on page 134.

Counting carbs is especially important if you want to be successful on a ketogenic diet, which demands a very high-fat intake but a low protein and carb intake. However, just wanting to lose weight and not exceeding 50 grams of carbs a day is a good way to get started. When you eat normally and healthily within the Green and Gold lists, you really don't need to count anything. Least of all any ratios, points or other diet-club type rituals – it's not natural, and it's not sustainable (and it's certainly not how to live LCHF).

There is no need to count fats or protein if you stick to the right proportions. Use a palm-sized portion of protein and thumb-sized portion of fat as a guideline. If you have to weigh, count and work out points, you will eventually rebel. LCHF is about freedom to enjoy the new-found delicious foods you can eat. Dump the diet mentality.

LEGUMES ARE PROTEIN AREN'T THEY?

We've been brainwashed into believing anything from the plant kingdom is better than anything from the animal kingdom, but this is not true. Animal protein and fat are far superior in every single way that matters – compared to what plants have to offer. Legumes comprise largely peanuts, peas and dried beans, and there are reasons why we suggest you don't eat legumes. They contain lectins and phytates (enzyme inhibitors) which prevent uptake of vital minerals. They can damage the gut lining, and even inhibit pancreatic enzyme function.

Legumes are also very high in carbs. Humans have digestive enzymes such as pepsin to break down proteins, amylase for starch digestion and trypsin is used in the digestion of protein – that's why eating foods which have trypsin inhibitors is damaging. Lentils have the highest level of trypsin inhibitors of all the legumes. But if you are on a low-carb lifestyle, all legumes are out of bounds so no need to worry.

WHY WE DON'T COUNT CALORIES.

History has proved to us that a calorie is not a calorie. Essentially a calorie is a measurement of energy, but that's really where it ends when it comes to effective weight loss. Food has a thermic effect on the body which is the number of calories used to digest and burn the food we have consumed. Protein, fat and carbohydrates are all burned as fuel in totally different ways. For example, protein uses around 25 per cent of its calories to process the food (which means it's very good for weight loss). Carbs use only five to 15 per cent of calories to process the food, and fat uses zero to five per cent. This doesn't mean fat is bad, it is more satiating, and you need much less. But carbs use very little of their calories to burn the food, so they are best at storing fat.

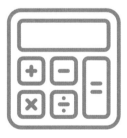

MEAT MYTHS.

With all the junk science around meat, let's clarify this right now: meat will not rot in your digestive tract, least of all in your colon, as some people may want you to think. If meat rots, then all the other food you eat does, too. If that did happen, we'd be like a huge walking compost heap.

When you eat protein, your stomach acid (which is close to battery acid), together with other digestive enzymes, is so strong, it breaks the protein into pieces and these are sent on to the small intestine where enzymes chop the pieces into single amino acids (building blocks). The fats are broken down into fatty acids, and from here, they get absorbed into the bloodstream – nothing is left to rot anywhere in the body. We don't have a stagnant system, it's moving all the time.

In fact, if anything is going to rot, it would be the indigestible plant matter from vegetables. Fibre isn't digested or broken down, and is evacuated from the body without being absorbed. However, while in the colon it gets fermented (this is a good thing, fermentation is not rotting) by the beneficial bacteria resident in the colon. The fermenting bacteria transform some of the fibre into beneficial compounds such as short-chain fatty acids like butyrate – which feeds the cells lining the colon. Fibre is the food of bacteria, and feeding them with the food they want is vital for good digestive health. Only plants rot in the colon, but not in the way we have been brainwashed to believe – they ferment.

Please get rid of the notion that meat causes cancer. Those same studies which looked at processed meat (which, it is agreed, probably would be instrumental in cancer) maligned good quality protein, but it is highly unlikely that pure pasture-fed meat would cause cancer. However, there does appear to be a strong correlation between processed meat and colon cancer. This is understandable if we look at the chemicals used.

Having said this, the way you cook your meat is of great importance, as this can impact health. There are compounds called heterocyclic amines and polycyclic aromatic hydrocarbons which form in overcooked meat. These have been linked to a possible cause of cancer in animals. To avoid this, never burn or blacken meat, and go more for lower temperature cooking rather than high-heat frying.

We are not designed to eat an exclusively plant-based diet: we were designed to eat meat, too. Our digestive system and our enzymes are uniquely designed for eating flesh. The digestive system of an herbivorous animal is completely different to that of a human being. The human has a stomach which produces hydrochloric acid to break down animal proteins, a long small intestine and a short colon. Human beings thrive best on a diet which is both plant and animal-based.

81

What about the myth about meat leaching calcium from your bones? How many times have we heard the unsubstantiated claim that meat causes osteoporosis? There is simply no scientific evidence to support this myth. On the contrary, overwhelming evidence points to the fact that a higher protein diet is linked to greatly improved bone density and a lower risk of osteoporosis and fractures in the elderly. Bone is made of collagen (a protein) which is impregnated with calcium, magnesium and phosphate salts.

HEART HEALTH MYTHS.

We have been deceived when it comes to what truly constitutes health. There are less-than healthy foods around (this is putting it mildly) which make people sick, and at best, offer them no nutritional benefit whatsoever. Why are these foods lauded as heart healthy?

We are being heavily influenced by some very slick and shrewd marketing strategies by food and drug companies to make their products appear as something worth purchasing, under the guise that they are somehow heart-healthy. From a promotional standpoint, this tactic is brilliant. Convince the consumer they need your product by underscoring all the supposed health benefits they will receive from purchasing and consuming it, and the money will roll in. Marketing is an amazing thing, especially to the uninformed.

On what basis are they staking their claim regarding something as being important when it comes to your cardiovascular health? How can you know if the product you are consuming is actually going to improve the health of your heart? Nobody asks these questions, and the public is extremely gullible. Yet nobody teaches us how to eat. How are we to know if we have never been taught good nutrition? Imagine yourself as a mum with a husband and kids, wanting to feed them healthily and doing your best, only to find out later that you've been conned into feeding them unhealthy food all along. Wouldn't you be angry?

What the industry calls heart-healthy generally equates to the following: the product in question is low in salt, fat and cholesterol, and high in so-called good fibre-based carbohydrates, or it tends to lower your LDL and total cholesterol. That's what constitutes a supposedly heart-healthy product.

Perhaps it's time to be more aware of creative advertising and educate yourself in proper nutrition to find out how unhealthy foods affect the body. The sad reality is that most of these products are probably doing more harm than good than you ever realised.

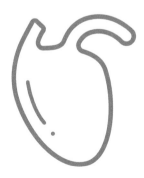

Chapter

03

SLEEP AND STRESS

THE SIGNIFICANCE OF HORMONES IN SLEEP.

A recent study in the journal *Nature Communications* found that if you deprive a person of sleep for a single night, increased cravings for junk food surface, together with a decreased ability to make sensible decisions about what kind of food to eat. Not getting enough regular, restorative sleep may prevent you from losing up to around eight kilograms a year. Hormones are responsible for these dietary fiascos, and without decent sleep you are much more likely to store fat than to burn it.

At least seven fat-regulating hormones are implicated when it comes to getting good quality sleep. Imbalances in these hormones may lead to weight gain, obesity and of course, other diseases.

1. **Leptin** – signals your brain that you've eaten enough and regulates your metabolism so that you burn fat when your body needs to. A study in *The Journal of Clinical Endocrinology and Metabolism* concluded that sleep duration influences leptin production which, in turn, adversely affects other hormones like cortisol and thyroid-stimulating hormones.

Researchers established that sleep modulates a major component of the neuroendocrine control of appetite.

2. **Ghrelin** – is the exact opposite of leptin, and tells your brain you are hungry and need to eat, your stomach even starts to rumble. A study in the *Journal of Sleep Research* showed being deprived of just one night of sleep increased ghrelin levels and hunger in healthy men of normal weight.

3. **Adiponectin** – is an anti-inflammatory hormone which helps predict cardiovascular risk and regulates several metabolic processes including fat oxidation (burning). Studies show optimum adiponectin levels can reduce your risk of insulin resistance and diabetes. A study in the journal *Physiology and Behavior* found reduced sleep decreases adiponectin production, which increased cardiovascular risk in women.

4. **Insulin** – elevated levels of this powerful fat-storing hormone will slam your fat-cell doors shut and lock them, storing fat and making it very difficult to release and be burned. Chronic sleep loss decreases insulin sensitivity, increases hunger and appetite and contributes to weight gain, insulin resistance and diabetes.

5. **Glucagon** – is the polar opposite of insulin, releasing fat from your fat cells to burn for energy. Studies show that too little sleep decreases the levels of circulating glucagon.

6. **Cortisol** – is one of the most important of our stress hormones. Raised levels seem to be something we all struggle with due to the stresses of just living on this planet. Our stress hormones can benefit us in the short term but, when chronically elevated, they will store fat and break down muscle tissue. Cortisol should

be at its highest level in the morning, tapering off as the day wears on.

7. **Growth hormone** – commonly known as the 'fountain of youth', this hormone is released during deep stage 4 sleep and boasts an enormous amount of benefits, such as muscle repair, increased energy and improved fat metabolism. Those who are light sleepers or wake several times during the night may not make optimal amounts of growth hormone.

Imagine that: having a good night's sleep actually helps you lose weight – what a pleasure. Many people exercise and eat well, but miss out on the third important pillar in the weight-loss triangle. They either don't sleep long enough, or their sleep quality is impaired. We need between six to eight hours a night, but too many people get less than five.

You may feel invincible with very little sleep and still perform well while you are young. But sleep is like a bank account. If you don't 'deposit' sleep into that account, you are not going to be able to find the health resources to draw on later. It's an inexorable depletion of the body systems which may take years off your life and add kilos to your waistline – kilos that are particularly hard to shift.

Losing sleep disturbs circadian rhythms, altering hunger and satiety hormones. Less sleep will also produce higher lipid levels. Getting less than five hours of sleep a night makes eating more pleasurable, so you tend to eat more. Sleeping more leads to eating less. Here's what you may experience with constant sleep deprivation of even an hour or two less a night:

· Increased cravings for sweet things and carbohydrates.
· It will take your body 40 per cent longer to regulate blood sugar than usual, especially after a high-carbohydrate meal.
· Your cortisol levels may increase.
· Insulin secretion and insulin response may decrease by up to 30 per cent.
· Leptin levels may decrease by 18 per cent or more.
· Ghrelin may increase by up to 28 per cent.

Whether you are a gym bunny or a couch potato, these symptoms can affect you if you don't get enough sleep. Too little sleep leads to reduced immune function, reduction in thyroid function, reduced ability to handle complex problems, memory loss, and many other symptoms. Russell Sanna of Harvard's Division of Sleep Medicine sums it up in a recent *Boston Globe* article: "Without adequate sleep, you get sick, fat and stupid."

STRESS.

Chronic stress activates an important hormone called cortisol, which stores fat. If you or anyone you know is thin yet still has that 'spare tyre' around the waist, chances are it's a cortisol tyre. Stress releases cortisol, giving you a middle-aged spread no matter how old you are. If your goal is weight loss, make stress management part of your plan. Sleep loss elevates cortisol levels the next night, and may cause metabolic and cognitive problems, and can significantly interrupt your sleep for the following night as well. Stress management is vital to health and wellness, and successful weight loss.

An interesting point here – some say the Mediterranean diet is the best for stress, but according to new thinking, it's in fact the daily siesta which is the secret to what is known as the Mediterranean diet.

TEN WAYS TO GET A GOOD NIGHT'S SLEEP

1. Plan to get enough sleep by going to bed at the same time each night.
2. Ensure you have a very dark bedroom. Use black-out curtains if you have a street light outside. This encourages the production of melatonin and serotonin.
3. Eat at least three hours prior to going to bed and don't snack in front of the TV.
4. Don't spend hours in front of the TV, computer or on a mobile phone or tablet before bed – wind down with a good book instead.
5. Put your mobile in another room and turn it off – it should not be in the same room – as radiation interrupts sleep. Remove any cordless phones, laptops or technology which could interfere with peaceful sleep.
6. Don't use an electric blanket, the conductive grid in the blanket upsets your own electric field and will interrupt your sleep – use a hot water bottle instead and wear socks and pyjamas if you are cold. Unromantic, but safe.

7. Use an old-fashioned non-electric clock – nothing electric or wireless as in a phone or digital clock.
8. Take as few drugs as possible – look for natural alternatives.
9. Try not to drink alcohol at night – it will interfere with your quality of sleep.
10. Have a well-ventilated room; being too hot or too cold also interferes with sleep quality.

The quality of your sleep is more important than the length. They are both vital, but when you do sleep, make sure it's a restorative, peaceful, deep sleep.

Try these things and throw in a few good stretches before climbing into bed. Sleep tight.

Chapter

03

THE THYROID GLAND

A dysfunctional thyroid may be a factor regarding weight gain in some people. T4 is a hormone made by the body, and converted into the more active hormone T3. (Please understand this is explained extremely simply to avoid getting too technical.) Thyroid stimulating hormone (TSH) tells the thyroid to make more T4. If your thyroid is under-active, the pituitary gland will continually send more TSH to stimulate the thyroid to make T4. Therefore, if TSH is high, the thyroid is generally under-active or hypothyroid; and if too low, you will have an over-active or hyperthyroid condition. Soya is often responsible for thyroid problems incidentally – another reason not to eat it.

Women in particular experience gut problems when they have raised thyroid antibodies, since the gut is intricately involved with the thyroid. Be aware that the thyroid responds adversely to poor diet and lifestyle; very often the culprits include gluten manifesting as either gluten intolerance or coeliac disease, which causes inflammation of the thyroid gland and even cancer. If your thyroid is inflamed, you could consider thyroid-supporting minerals such as selenium, zinc and iron, but never take supplemental iron without having a blood test (ferritin) to establish whether you need it.

SYMPTOMS OF A SLUGGISH THYROID.

If you suspect you suffer from hypothyroidism, you may have some of the following symptoms:

- Unexplained weight gain
- Fatigue and lack of stamina
- Depression
- A swelling in your neck (goitre)
- Dry skin and hair
- Hair loss
- Intolerance to cold even on warm days
- Voice may get lower (not always)
- Regular constipation
- Thinning or disappearance of the hair on your lower legs
- Decrease in the hairs on the outer third of your eyebrows
- Puffy eyes in the morning
- Feeling of tightness around throat, sore throat, even difficulty swallowing

Please note: There are many other conditions that may cause these symptoms; however, when taken together, they can often point to hypothyroidism. Whenever you are in doubt, please contact a qualified health professional or medical doctor.

Hyperthyroidism is the opposite of hypothyroidism, and manifests with sweating, rapid heartbeat, anxiety, tremors, fatigue (common to both conditions), insomnia, weight loss and protruding eyes. See your doctor if you suspect you have either of these conditions. You will need to support your thyroid gland with the mineral selenium, essential for effecting the conversion from T4 to T3.

Further thyroid support

- Remove soya, grains, sugar, seed oils and all junk food.
- Remove 'deadly nightshade' vegetables (potatoes, aubergines, peppers and tomatoes, even cayenne) as these may, in some instances, contribute to autoimmune thyroid conditions.
- Remove dairy products except for butter.
- Often nuts and seeds are problematic.
- Remove artificial sweeteners.
- Drink homemade bone broth daily for beneficial minerals.
- Coconut oil is well known as a powerful thyroid support, and it helps weight loss as it contains medium chain fatty acids and lauric acid.
- Get to sleep early at night.
- Manage stress.
- Do gentle exercise.

Thyroid-supporting supplements

Vitamin C – take one to two grams with each meal.
Vitamin D – transports thyroid hormone into the cells.
Selenium – converts T4 to the more active T3 hormone. Take 200 micrograms per day.
Probiotics and probiotic foods – the thyroid like everything else, is all about gut health.

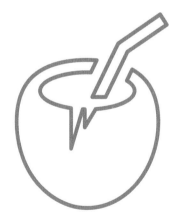

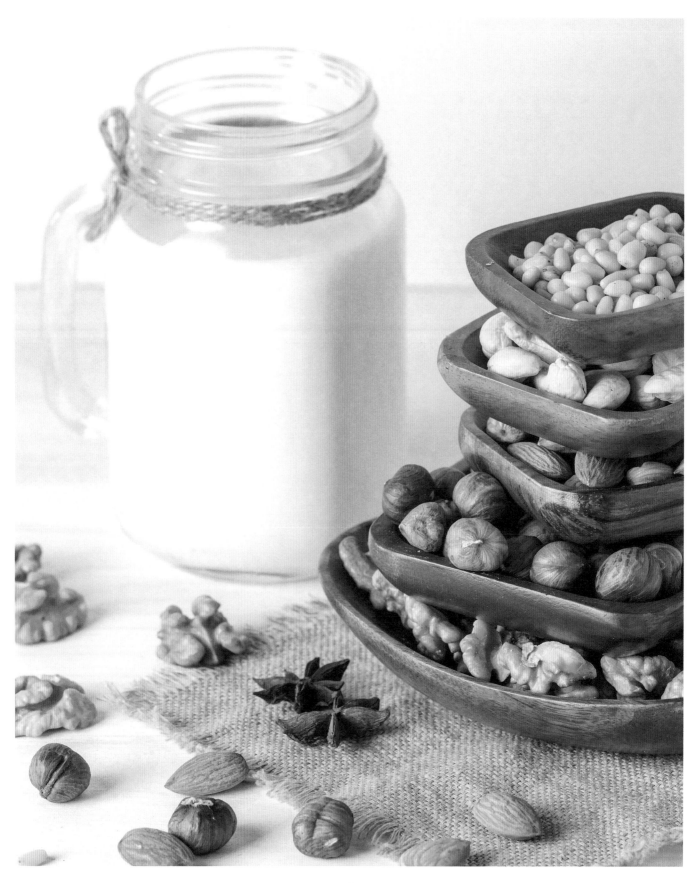

Chapter

03

GREY AREAS

THE GREY LIST.

These are foods which are considered grey area foods, mainly because they react differently in people. Essentially, they will often prevent weight loss, may be harmful, may cause severe allergies, bloating and discomfort – even though some of them are technically low-carb. If your weight loss has plateaued or you have health issues, it may be worth avoiding them. Some are still wholefoods, others are not, yet permitted in small amounts.

Grey list items:

- Alcohol
- Beans
- Chocolate
- Dairy products
- Every type of cream (heavy, pouring, whipping)
- Fruit
- Goat's cheese
- Goat's milk
- Kefir (dairy)
- Kombucha
- Nut and seed flours
- Nuts and seeds
- Peas

DAIRY.

The first truly grey area is dairy products. Dairy is universally loved, but it has no fibre, is very easy to overeat, and it's high in calories, fat-building hormones, sugar (lactose) and is an insulinogenic food – dairy must be limited or avoided. You could be lactose intolerant or have problems with casein or whey present (milk proteins), and then there is the spectre of Insulin-like Growth Factor No. 1 (IGF#1).

One thing is certain, dairy can put the brakes on weight loss. It raises blood sugar and insulin, which is not great if you are insulin resistant or diabetic. Dairy appears to cause a disproportionate spike in insulin levels. Cream and cheese may be slightly less problematic, but will still cause weight gain; cream especially should be limited. Milk and most yoghurts appear to have an even greater insulin response than white bread. Caution is advised.

NUTS AND SEEDS.

Too many nuts and seeds may cause weight gain. They are higher in carbs than you realise, and are fairly high in pro-inflammatory omega-6 fatty acids. Both omega-3 and omega-6 fatty acids are essential to life, but we tend to get far more omega-6 than omega-3 fats in our diet, which creates an imbalance. This imbalance causes inflammation, which can be a direct cause of disease and weight gain.

The current low-carb craze has everyone baking furiously with seed and nut flours. They imagine they can eat cakes, muffins and pizza bases made from seed and nut flours with impunity. Not so – they must be eaten frugally.

Nuts and seeds, like legumes, have enzyme inhibitors which prevent absorption of valuable minerals, and they possess anti-nutrients which steal nutrients rather than provide them. By activating nuts and seeds, the phytic acid and lectins are rendered harmless making them tastier, more nutritious and safer to eat (see section on activating nuts, page 158). However, I still recommend you eat them sparingly.

CHOCOLATE.

Commercial, sugary chocolate can be pretty harmful if you read the labels – they contain a brew of ingredients you wouldn't normally consider eating. Remember this is not a necessary food, it's an indulgence. Please eat responsibly. Aim for a

sugar-free chocolate that doesn't have a list of hazardous ingredients.

ALCOHOL.

Most people throw up their hands in horror at the thought of stopping alcohol, but the fact remains that it is a depressant, a liver toxin and certainly not an essential wholefood. Alcohol is not part of a healthy diet. Excess, as we know, leads to a fatty liver which is the first step to cirrhosis, diabetes, heart disease and cancer. You can build alcohol into your diet if you drink moderately – the choice is yours. You may argue it's low-carb, yes, but remember, it's about much more than just the carbs and that's why it is a grey area.

CAFFEINE.

Coffee and caffeinated teas can be fabulously soothing, and even healthy in some cases. But if you find yourself needing many cups a day to remain focused, it may be time to cut down. Stimulants like caffeine elicit a strong insulin response in some people, even if unsweetened and black. In others, caffeine may prevent weight loss and lead to poor quality sleep, which in itself can prevent weight loss; while still others appear to thrive on a daily cuppa. Enjoy caffeine frugally, don't overdo it. If you have adrenal issues, stick to Swiss water decaf coffee and herbal teas.

FRUIT.

Fruit is certainly whole, real food – and may be eaten moderately by Paleo enthusiasts and those wishing to only eat real food. The trouble is fruit is high in sugar (fructose), which in excess will lead to weight gain, and even very serious blood sugar dysregulation in sensitive individuals, insulin resistance and even diabetes. Eat fruit sparingly: it's nature's form of confectionary. Daily excess, especially on an empty stomach, is a mistake.

BEANS AND PEAS.

Legumes have anti-nutrients, protease inhibitors, saponins and a host of other compounds which should make them out of bounds on a healthy low-carb diet, due to the effect they have on our digestive health. So what about peas and beans? Whole peas are still legumes. However, if you eat the flat pods before the peas form, as in mangetout, this is acceptable. What you are eating is the fibrous pod, not the 'seed', which is the pea inside. The fibrous green pod would be classed as a wholefood – but if you eat the formed peas you are eating legumes.

Green beans are legumes too, however, due to the exceptionally tiny seeds inside, most experts do not consider them to be problematic, especially if it doesn't form a large part of the diet. If you are trying to stay low-carb or have a gut permeability problem, or if you bloat after peas and beans, you are not tolerating the enzyme inhibitors well. Although higher in carbs in the form of sucrose, it's about more than the carbs present in the food. Enzyme inhibitors bind to minerals in our food, preventing absorption. Eaten regularly, these may lead to mineral deficiencies of extremely important minerals like calcium, magnesium and zinc, as well as others. Beans and peas are still legumes, botanically speaking.

The father of modern Paleo, Loren Cordain, slates peas and beans out of hand for their anti-nutrient properties. However, he says that green beans are probably a better bet than any other legumes. Because they contain such a tiny seed, and because you can cook them, they are definitely more acceptable than peas. With only seven grams per 100 grams, with 2.7 grams of that being fibre, they have a net carb count of 4.3 grams per 100 grams, (scraping through onto the Green list). If you absolutely must have baby green beans, cook them well, and eat them infrequently.

Nutritional analyses online are not always that helpful for those wanting absolute clarity – peas have different carb counts depending on which source you use – is it 19 grams per 100 grams or seven grams per 100 grams – who do you believe? They are *still* legumes, and are not particularly rich in nutrients, so avoiding them for the most part is best. There are plenty of other non-legume foods to eat.

Have a look at Loren's article, "Beans and Legumes: Do they Adhere to Paleo?" for more clarity (see the Bibliography on page 249).

04

LET'S GO LCHF

When weight loss is achieved, you do not put carbohydrates back into the diet. That will reintroduce the craving and addiction for carbohydrates and sweets. What we do to put a halt to the weight loss is to increase the protein.

– Dr Richard K Bernstein

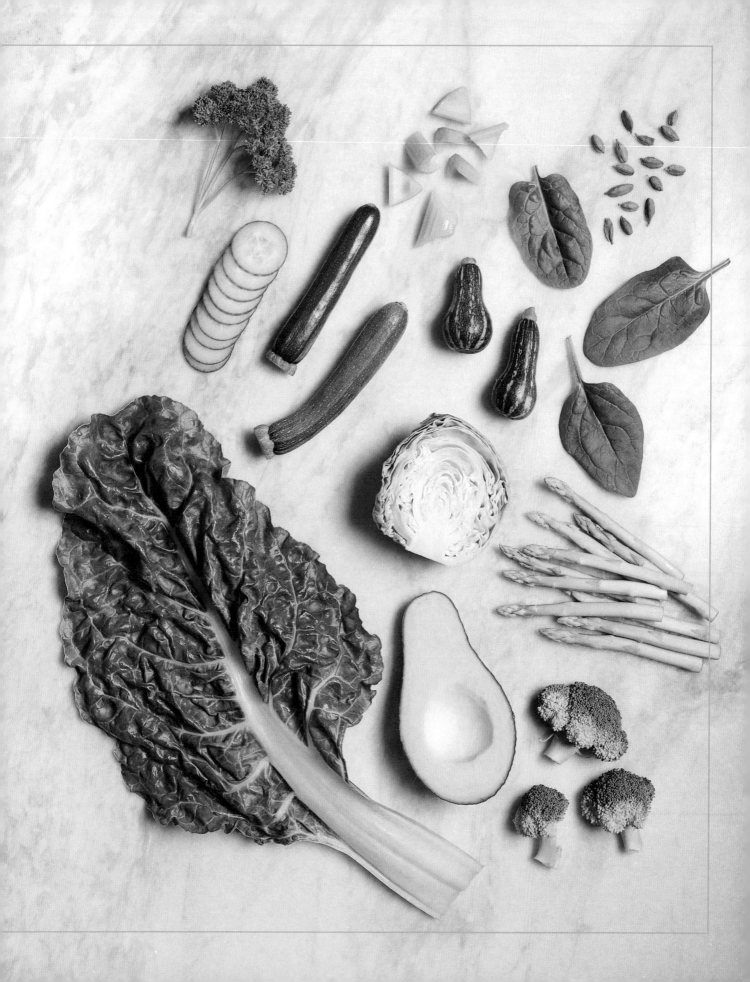

Chapter

04

OVERVIEW OF POPULAR LOW-CARB DIETS

There are dozens of low-carb diets around – here are just a few of the better-known ones.

ATKINS DIET.

In 1972, Dr Atkins published his famous book, *Dr Atkins' Diet Revolution*, in which he outlined his four-phase programme, starting with a very low-carbohydrate intake and ended up adding back quite a lot of the foods which were responsible for the initial problem. Atkins fell prey to the 'needs' of Americans by including plenty of puddings, snacks, processed foods and ice cream into the carbohydrate allowance. I don't believe these foods are helpful to either health or weight loss, as most of them are not nourishing and they certainly are not real food. Fat is not restricted in the diet, and he recommends supplements.

BANTING.

The term "Banting" was resurrected in 2013 with the release of the red book in South Africa. It describes a particular type of low-carb eating that follows the Swedish version of LCHF with a strong emphasis on real food. It recommends avoiding junk food and processed food, and advocates a return to the way our grandparents ate. It eschews the use of grains, sugar, seed oils, processed food, fizzy drinks, artificial sweeteners and chemicals, and relies on grass-fed, organic food: meat, eggs, fish, vegetables and healthy fats. It is a higher healthy fat, moderate protein and low-carb diet. The idea hinges on eating wholesome, close-to-the-earth food, and cooking it from scratch with tender loving care. A core pillar of the paradigm is to control insulin by regulating the amount of carbohydrates eaten.

DUKAN DIET.

Developed by Dr Pierre Dukan, this is a no fun diet as it's a high-protein, low-carb and low-fat eating plan, and may leave you hungry and obsessing over food. It seems wholly unsustainable due to being both low-carb and low-fat, and relatively high-protein. Without fat, satiety is not reached. Vegetables are restricted and there are protein-only days where no vegetables are permitted. Dukan embraces phases much like Atkins did, and oats are permitted, flying in the face of the generally accepted no-grain philosophy of low-carb living.

KETOGENIC DIET.

The ketogenic diet (often called just 'keto') is a nutritional approach that aims to induce ketosis by restricting the amount of carbohydrates to a minimum. You could call it extreme LCHF. It is high-fat, fairly low-protein and very low-carb. Ketosis is a natural state that occurs once the body starts burning fat for fuel instead of carbohydrates. The usual ketogenic range for most people is 20 to 30 grams net carbs a day, although highly active people can go up to 50 grams and remain in ketosis. Ketosis was the very successful standard treatment for epilepsy prior to the advent of anticonvulsant drugs.

PALEO/PRIMAL/ ANCESTRAL/CAVEMAN/ STONE AGE DIETS.

I believe Paleo is the sanest and best lifestyle after the stricter Banting approach (in fact, it may be better in many ways for people who don't fare well on Banting) as it is based on wholefood, grass-fed meat, wild caught fish, organic veggies and fruit, and old-fashioned cooking methods. No chemicals, junk food or processed foods are permitted. Because the diet excludes grains, dairy and seed oils, it is by default a low-carb diet. It does allow fruit and small amounts of natural sugars like honey and some dried fruit. No refined sugar, legumes or chemicals are permitted.

The Primal diet is very similar, the main proponent of this being the American Mark Sisson. He emphasises the importance of sleep, play and high-intensity exercise. All these diets are modelled similarly on the Paleo diet.

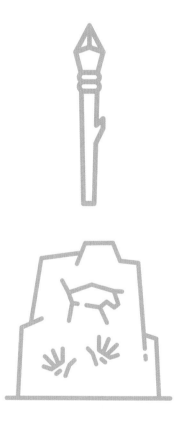

Chapter

04

LCHF VERSUS PACEO

Paleo has swept the world. In fact, in 2013, 'Paleo' was one of the most frequently searched words online, and awareness has only increased since then. The other reason Paleo is popular is that it allows a wider variety of food, such as some starchy vegetables, fruit and honey. Not that these will help with weight loss, but they are there to indulge in occasionally if you are following a Paleo approach.

There are subtle differences between the LCHF lifestyle and the Paleo lifestyle. Common to both are:

- Pasture-fed meats and eggs, wild game and poultry
- No grains
- No refined sugar
- No legumes or pulses (soya, lentils, etc)
- No seed oils
- No microwaves
- No processed food
- Real food only
- No plastic

The last four items on the above list seem to have been forgotten by some people following a LCHF lifestyle these days, but Paleo is generally pretty rigid on these points. We need to understand it's not about eating rubbish or processed versions of LCHF food. It's not about convenience. Many people have neglected to see that this is about real food, not processed food. We hope to remind you about this in this book.

The Paleo movement is very focused when it comes to purity, even though there are those in the LCHF community who seem to have lost their way, many reverting to the seed oils and processed foods we have tried so hard to get away from – it's these we believe made us sick and overweight in the first place. It's our fervent desire in this book to make it clear that a low-carb lifestyle should always be about purity, single-ingredient foods, and loving care put into cooking from scratch. Low-carb living should never be about convenience. Our obsession as a society for convenience has lined many pockets of entrepreneurs, no doubt, but it has done nothing for our health. We need to ensure we are choosing quality wholefood over processed convenient food, even if it claims to be low-carb (or sprinkled with pixie dust).

No one size fits all. You may find that LCHF works perfectly well for you all of the time; you may wish to stay in ketosis or never try it at all; or you may find that after a while it stops working. For still others, the Paleo lifestyle seems to be ideal.

I have noticed in the past year or so that people are veering away from LCHF to a more Paleo-based lifestyle for various reasons. One could be partly due to the confusion created by social media 'advisors' – conflicting advice always causes confusion. We hope to straighten out some of the confusion in this book.

I'm amazed at the fervour with which LCHF adherents have embarked on this journey – some for the good, some sadly not so much. It seems all of a sudden anything goes, and some nasties have made a comeback including the foods which caused the problem in the first place, such as seed oils and gluten – which is so sad. The old culprits we have moved away from will present the same result sooner or later; it's just a matter of time. Please read labels if you must buy food with a label on it. Regardless of who endorses products for marketing advantage, this is about you and your body – read the labels to be better informed.

So let's look at what Paleo enthusiasts advocate.

PALEO.

Paleo makes allowance for the following, which Banting does not:

- Various types of natural sweeteners, from coconut sugar to molasses and honey (all in small amounts)
- Tapioca flour, arrowroot flour – again, in small amounts
- Dried fruit in limited quantities
- Fresh fruit in limited quantities
- All vegetables usually, even high-carb ones, in small amounts

Paleo followers will eat only:

- Grass-fed meats, wild-caught fish and food as pure as possible
- Organic food
- Single-ingredient foods to be cooked from scratch
- Nuts and seeds only in activated form

Paleo does not include:

- Alcohol
- Anything bottled, cured or processed
- Artificial sweeteners
- Cereals
- Chemicals, preservatives, colourants, anything fake
- Dairy products (sometimes including butter, though that is changing)
- Grains
- Legumes and pulses, beans, peas (including all forms of peas as well as snow peas and sugar snap peas), beans, lentils, alfalfa, carob, soya, lupins and peanuts
- Potatoes
- Processed foods
- Refined sugar
- Seed oils
- Soft drinks, fizzy drinks and fruit juice

- Soya (in case you don't realise, it's a legume)
- Sweets of any kind
- Very high-carb veggies (mostly)

Modern Paleo food consists of:

- Animal protein derived from any organic/free range sources of beef, lamb, rabbit, poultry and pork
- Eggs – from hens that roam free – chicken, duck, etc.
- Fat – any animal fat, from bacon to duck fat, ghee, lard or tallow, with restraint
- Fermented foods made at home to colonise and improve gut health
- Fish and seafood – only wild-caught, never farmed
- Fruit – as with vegetables, local, in season, organic, and not too much
- Grass-fed butter (only – not commercial)
- Honey or maple syrup – just a little, or stevia
- Nuts – all nuts in activated form but not peanuts (these are legumes)
- Oils – olive, avocado, coconut, macadamia nut and other nut oils like walnut
- Seeds – most seeds, but never seed oils
- Vegetables in abundance, but they need to be local and organic where possible
- And lastly, it's *quality over quantity*

While Paleo is said to be based on how our ancestors supposedly ate in the Palaeolithic era, nobody knows for sure what people ate millions of years ago. Whether you believe in creation or evolution, the fact is we need to know how to eat today. So while we may not always agree with the roots of where Paleo came from, we absolutely love the pure philosophy of good old-fashioned food and traditional cooking methods. In fact, our diet has changed almost completely over the last 60 to 100 years, so why fuss about thousands of years?

Even just 100 years ago there was no refrigeration, no supermarkets with fruit juice and ready meals, no microwaves, and virtually no cancer or obesity. What we should be asking ourselves is what are we going to do about all this *now*? Paleo is not about counting anything and not about excess, it is a moderate lifestyle.

The Paleo model says we need to eat what we can hunt (not literally, but what can be hunted or raised humanely for food); grow and eat in terms of vegetables; pick as in fruits; catch in terms of fish; or glean as in eggs laid by chickens or collecting honey. Animal protein is fine in all its forms, fruits and berries are good in moderation, nuts and seeds (activated is best) in moderation, with perhaps a little honey on occasion. Paleo is truly about real food in its most natural form. What came to be known as 'Banting' should be too, but for many it is no longer a pure discipline.

Truth be told, 90 per cent of the international LCHF community is Paleo, and for most, it is much easier to sustain than a stricter approach. The trick is that you need to ensure that the model you adopt does in fact work for you.

With Paleo, you get to have a little fruit, a little honey (if you so choose), but you also avoid the perils of grains, dairy, damaged fats, legumes and processed food. It would seem then that Paleo could either be a viable alternative to the stricter approach, or a natural transition once your goal weight is reached. It's an individual choice.

The Paleo lifestyle is neither fat-heavy nor low-fat, although it is very pro-natural fat. Paleo advocates do not do fat bombs, Bulletproof coffee overdosing or strive for huge amounts of fat. It's just about eating real food from the land in the most natural form possible. The food variety is greater and it's much more relaxed.

What many people find helpful is getting to their goal weight on a stricter low-carb programme like LCHF, and then moving naturally into Paleo. You will still eliminate grain, of course, and many of the things you are used to avoiding, but the shift in focus may be a welcome change in some cases. If you have serious blood sugar issues, you may need to continue to avoid fruit and foods that spike your blood sugars. You are not required to perform intellectual suicide.

Imagine living on a farm with everything you need – from beehives to cows, sheep, chickens, eggs, a lake or sea nearby with fish, a few pigs, ducks, and a large organic vegetable garden – that is a Paleo lifestyle. You would work the land yourself and eat from your own abundance. You'd also enjoy plenty of fresh air, restful sleep (no microwaves or TV), good conversation, sun, fun and friends. This is the Paleo lifestyle in a nutshell.

Today we suffer diseases of affluence such as cardiovascular problems, diabetes, obesity, Alzheimer's and dozens of other dread diseases. Modern man has too much stress, too little sleep, shocking dietary habits, and a sedentary lifestyle – all of which end in ill health. There are too many drugs, and nobody's teaching society how to eat apart from 'Big Food'. Years ago, before fast food surfaced, you never saw an overweight person – if you are 45 or over, you'll probably remember people in your childhood all being slim. Seeing an overweight person today is the norm. How did we get here?

It's said that the children of this generation will not live as long as their parents. In a day when medical technology and drugs are able to keep people alive much longer than they'd have done naturally, the children are already sick before puberty. What hope do they have?

We have to do something about getting back to eating healthy, real food. There's no other alternative. In fact, most people end up going Paleo due to ill health, regain their health and are converts for life.

MODERN PALEO.

I recommend something we call 'modern' Paleo. It's not pretending to eat what we imagine people ate many millions of years ago, nor is it ridiculous. It's being sensible, and doing the best we can in a less-than-perfect world. We can all avoid the central aisle of the supermarket, and buy wholefood even if we are too lazy or don't have space to grow food ourselves. To some degree we all have access to healthier meat, fats and vegetables.

There really is no excuse. Modern man can still be a hunter-gatherer (which isn't Paleo, but this is modern Paleo); he now has the advantage of the internet to 'hunt' for information on where to find things, and then 'gather' them up, either by buying them online or seeking out the source.

Some people do a mixture of Paleo and strict low-carb, but as there is no one-size-fits-all solution; you need to find what suits you. Some Paleo and Primal people eat a little fermented dairy, others have only butter, no other dairy, and still others consume no dairy at all. Perhaps years ago, before we started introducing hormones and growth promoters to dairy, before we pasteurised and homogenised milk, less people were intolerant to it.

Years ago, we also ate less dairy. Yoghurt was homemade, cream carefully and lovingly scraped from the top of the milk from hand-milked cows – today, everything's industrialised. Our bodies are more sensitive due to the drugs, chemicals, junk and stress we are subjected to – can we even handle dairy anymore? Having said that, there are raw cheeses that some Paleo followers

eat, and these can be very nutritious if you are not intolerant to dairy.

In essence, Paleo works because it focuses only on real food, never on processed foods, and thereby many sugars, preservatives and unnatural substances are by default removed from the diet. If it's in a packet or a bottle in a store, you can safely say it's not Paleo.

Aren't you amazed at how few people worry about pizza, muffins and soft drinks being unhealthy, yet they attack the low-carb lifestyle? Somehow eating piles of grain and sugar is never considered unsafe, and you are deemed to be heading into dangerous territory health-wise the moment you remove them.

LOSING WEIGHT ON A PALEO PROGRAMME.

You will still lose weight if you follow these guidelines sensibly. You're cutting out dairy, alcohol, grains, refined and processed food, and are eating just natural, real food, so you have an advantage already. Very often, just transitioning from a normal diet to this way of eating is enough to bring about permanent change. Provided you are not gung-ho with honey, fruit or starchy veggies, you have a fighting chance of making Paleo work for you.

Eating good food is key to both health and weight loss. A well-nourished body and a healthy liver will enable much faster weight loss. The nutrient-dense nature of Paleo living and its balanced lifestyle are conducive to good health in every way that matters.

Paleo principles extend to the rest of your lifestyle, not only food – there is an emphasis on exercise, relaxation, fun, family, not too much electromagnetic field (EMF) exposure and general balance. It is a very holistic approach.

By eating high-quality food, you bring down inflammation in the body, a very real cause of weight gain. It will help to balance hormones too, which are fundamental to losing weight. You will, in effect, provide your body with the wherewithal to be healthy enough to lose weight.

IN SUMMARY.

For many, Paleo will be the most sustainable lifestyle choice long term. If you are not obese or hypersensitive, Paleo would be an excellent option. If you are diabetic, maybe it's best to be stricter due to the fruit and high-carb veggies allowed; yet there are many diabetics who thrive on this programme.

If there is one glaring flaw in Paleo, it is the possibility of over-consuming sweet fruits, honey, dried fruit and starchy vegetables. Yet, this doesn't seem to be the case most of the time, as most Paleo followers realise that these foods are to be used frugally. It is more attractive to sweeten your food with a natural sweetener like raw honey (if it's needed, very occasionally) than any other kind of sweetener, but this needs to be strictly controlled.

Chapter

04

THE LCHF CODE

Study the previous chapters to get a feel for what you should and should not include in your diet. Getting started is not difficult.

Remove the following from your diet:

· Grains
· Sugar
· Seed oils
· Legumes
· Processed food of every sort

Just eat real, fresh food. This is a great start.

Have a look at the Green and Gold lists, and stick to these two lists initially (maybe forever).

GETTING STARTED.

· Remember first and foremost, this is about being healthy, eating real food, and feeling fabulous. Weight loss is a bonus.
· Start the day with a good breakfast of protein (eggs), fat (done in butter) and something green (like watercress, spinach or asparagus); add bacon, tomato or mushrooms, etc. (What's life without bacon anyway?)

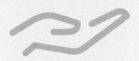

PORTION SIZE GUIDE PER MEAL

2 cupped hands =
1 portion of leafy salad greens (raw)

A fist size =
portion of Green list vegetables (raw)

Thumb size =
a fat serving or a serving of cheese

Palm of hand without fingers =
serving of animal protein (red meat, chicken or fish – can have a little more fish)

- Eat only when you are hungry. Do not eat meals out of habit.
- Drink plenty of pure water. Half an hour before a meal, have a glass of water. Add a spoon of apple cider vinegar in for extra probiotic benefits.
- The brain often registers thirst as hunger: drink a glass of water before snacking.
- Exercise is a great stress reliever. You may not burn off a lot of fat while exercising, but building muscle from exercise is helpful, as resting muscle continues to burn fat 24 hours a day.
- Don't have second helpings. If you are desperate for seconds, force yourself to wait 20 minutes. You won't be hungry after a while.
- Increase the fibre content of your diet – it will keep you full for longer. Processed food doesn't do that. Vegetables are a great source of fibre. If you need more (as some people get constipated), then psyllium husk fibre is a great low-carb, healthy alternative to laxatives, and will cause neither weight gain nor dependence. Please make sure that you drink more water though – whenever fibre is increased, water intake must be increased.
- Just drop the carbohydrates now once and for all – no more bread, pasta, rice and potatoes. And no more excuses!

Make sure you are eating correctly and understand the difference between the foods you should be eating and those you shouldn't. You will need to make sure you are getting enough protein and fat primarily, and not overdoing any of the starchy vegetables – watch out for 'carb-creep' where carbs slip into your diet. Perhaps the biggest hurdle of all is avoiding eating constant treats to replace the treats you were used to before LCHF – they will derail you, even if they are LCHF.

AVOID

- **Sugar:** Soft drinks, fruit juices, agave, fructose, sweets, ice cream, cake, etc. Sugar is addictive, insulinogenic, inflammatory and obesogenic.
- **Grains:** Wheat, spelt, barley, rice and rye, all breads and pastas, rolls, croissants – anything made from a grain or grain flour or containing any gluten – they damage the gut lining.
- **Trans fats:** Hydrogenated or partially hydrogenated oils are toxic.
- **All vegetable/seed oils:** Cottonseed, soyabean, sunflower, grapeseed, corn, safflower, canola, flaxseed, hemp – these are harmful fats.

- **Artificial sweeteners:** Acesulfame K, cyclamates, aspartame, saccharin and sucralose. Although calorie-free, studies show a massive association with insulin resistance and obesity. Insulin and leptin signalling is significantly disturbed and inhibited in the brain by the chemicals in artificial sweeteners. Use stevia, erythritol or xylitol instead.
- **Diet, lite, fat-free and low-fat products:** Choose full-fat options as low-fat foods are highly processed and loaded with sugar and/or artificial sweeteners. Diet foods are almost always processed.
- **Commercial, processed food:** Nothing out of a box or wrapper. This is called junk food.

EAT

- **Meat/poultry:** Beef, lamb, pork, chicken and game. Grass-fed is best.
- **Fish:** Salmon, trout, haddock, herring, etc. Eat wild-caught, not farmed. Eat fatty fish with teeth (not swordfish, due to high mercury levels).
- **Eggs:** Pasture-raised if possible.
- **Vegetables:** Spinach, broccoli, cauliflower and all those on the Green list.
- **Fruits:** A few berries.
- **Nuts and seeds:** See the lists for the best nut and seed choices. Activated nuts and seeds are preferred.

- **High-fat dairy:** Cheese, butter, double cream, Greek yoghurt. Avoid if weight loss is slowing down; avoid milk anyway. It is obesogenic and insulinogenic.
- **Fats and oils:** Butter, lard, duck fat, olive oil, coconut oil, tallow, goose fat, macadamia oil and avocado oil.

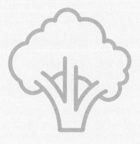

SHOPPING.

Shopping on a LCHF diet should not be difficult at all. In essence, you will want to take with you a list of foods that are permitted, and perhaps a short list of those you aren't certain of (for example, carrots are a little higher in carbs – and you may want only one carrot for a broth, not an entire bunch) so that you know how many carbs to work towards. The main things to remember are as follows:

1. Buy fresh, single-ingredient foods wherever possible such as green leafy vegetables, whole cabbage, nut and seed flours if you wish to make low-carb bread – don't buy ready-made anything. If you want tomato sauce, buy the fresh ingredients and make it yourself.

2. There are times you will be a little stuck. For example, if you wish to make tomato sauce, you may need some organic tomato paste – this is where you will have to read labels very carefully to ensure there is nothing nasty in it, and there is no sugar, corn starch, seed oils, wheat, etc. You want very pure ingredients. My advice is everything fresh, and everything made from scratch. When you absolutely cannot do that, get the purest tinned or boxed version you can.

3. Essentially avoid anything premixed, premade or made for you. All processed, prepared and 'dead' food should be excluded. This lifestyle is about returning to the way we ate 100 years ago when you did it yourself from scratch`– there were no bottled sauces! Avoid the middle aisles – stick to the living aisles where there is fresh food, meat, chicken, butter and eggs – the rest are the 'cemetery' aisles where all the dead food lies.

Tips for shopping

- Have a list of items you need and don't deviate.
- Stick to the outside perimeter of the store. This includes the fruit and vegetable section, the butchery and sometimes the dairy deli. Avoid the 'dead food' in the centre aisles.
- If the food has to sell itself on the packaging, don't buy it.
- If it has a long list of ingredients, don't buy it.
- Leave foods that contain unnatural preservatives alone; you want your food to wilt and die, not live in the fridge or pantry forever.
- Buy fresh ingredients and assemble foods, sauces and gravies yourself.
- Don't buy oils and fats in plastic, including salad dressings. Make your own. Read sauce ingredients carefully – or better yet, don't buy pre-made sauces at all.
- Buy meat unmarinated and fresh. Buy organic or pasture-fed meat that is also hormone-free whenever possible. If you purchase frozen meat, check that no brine has been added that contains sugar.
- Buy fresh herbs and vegetables. If you buy dried herbs, check the label first. Avoid the following: irradiated spices, maize, breadcrumbs – these are often in our dried spices. If buying frozen vegetables, check the labelling and avoid brine and sugar.
- Buy free-range eggs wherever possible.
- Buy best quality butter, extra virgin cold-pressed olive oil and extra virgin cold-pressed coconut oil.
- Be mindful of products that proclaim to be Banting-friendly or make any play on the words to suggest being low-carb. These may

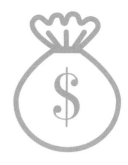

include so-called LCHF products, some low-carb products, and other such names.

- Gluten-free products are not always low-carb, but low-carb should always be gluten-free.
- Learn to read labels for substances you may not wish to put into your body.

AFFORDABLE LCHF.

There is the perception that LCHF is a rich man's diet and is unaffordable for the majority of the population. This has come about because people believe that to start this lifestyle they need to stock up on all the expensive products that are used to produce replica breads and treats. But there is no need to use any of the expensive products such as nut flours and sweeteners to follow a LCHF lifestyle, and excluding them will lead to faster weight loss.

The other misconception is the amount of protein required. Don't confuse LCHF with a high-protein diet, and think that the vast quantities of meat make it unaffordable. (Offal is a wonderfully nutritious source of protein instead of muscle meats, and extremely inexpensive for those trying to budget – we've included some good offal recipes in this book.) Most people who start LCHF may even need to decrease their protein intake – this is a moderate protein diet. Sticking to protein, vegetables and healthy fats will result in a lower grocery bill. No more cold drinks, biscuits or commercial bread. An added bonus is that you will end up eating smaller, less-frequent meals, and not be hungry all the time.

Tips for making LCHF really affordable

- Stick to seasonal vegetables instead of out-of-season ones at inflated prices just because they are on the Green list. Use what is available, and buy fresh, not frozen.
- Plant a vegetable garden. Spinach, lettuce and herbs are all easy to grow, as are many other vegetables.
- Buy cheaper, fatty cuts of meat, and cook them well. Brisket is cheaper than rump steak and far tastier.
- Liver, tripe, trotters, marrow bones, and all other parts of the animal that you may have been reluctant to eat, are loaded with nutrition – more so than muscle meat – and are extremely inexpensive.
- Save chicken bones to turn into a bone broth, or buy bones to make broth, which will add nutrition to everything you cook.
- Make stews with lots of vegetables, a little protein and bone broth. This is really good for you.
- Buy fat from your butcher – lamb, pork or beef – and render it down to make lard or tallow. Place it in a pan in the oven, or heat it in a pot on the stove. The crispy bits you are left with make delicious snacks, and the wonderful liquid can be poured into a glass jar. When set, you can use it for cooking later. It's very affordable, and a fantastic source of fat for cooking vegetables, or frying meat.
- Eggs are a wonder food, inexpensive and full of nutrition. Eggs with leftover vegetables make a great way to start the day, eat them any way

you like, any time of day. Take hard boiled eggs to work to eat cold.

· Tinned pilchards in brine are also a good source of protein (not in tomato sauce).

· Make your own cream cheese from maas. It's very easy; line a colander with muslin cloth and place the colander over a bowl. Pour in the maas, two litres makes just over 600 grams of cheese. Let it drain for 24 hours. The cream cheese is then ready to use. You can use the remaining liquid, called whey, to add to soups and stews; it is very nutritious.

· Don't get caught by cheap coffee, it often contains sugar or sugar substitutes. Rather buy a more expensive pure coffee, and drink less. Don't use instant coffee.

· Try to cut out all sweeteners – xylitol will push up the cost of your grocery bill.

· Stick to basics; get the majority of your fat from lard and tallow. Butter and coconut oil will be the pricier items in your grocery basket, but they are worth getting – they'll last a while.

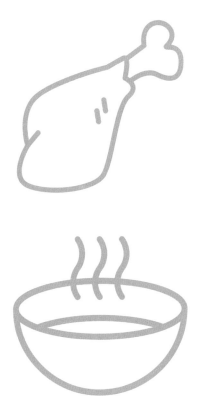

Chapter

04

LOSING WEIGHT ON LCHF

Sometimes during a weight-loss programme, your weight loss seems to stall, and there are many reasons for this. Firstly, don't expect to keep losing weight at a rapid rate on LCHF; your weight loss will slow down as you get close to your goal weight. However, it could be that you are doing something wrong which is causing you to stop losing, or even to put on weight. Please remember though, we are not machines, we're human beings: complex, complicated, beautiful creatures with a variety of different reasons for why things don't work. We need a certain amount of nutrients to function properly – this is one area you might want to look at – but there are dozens of possibilities. Here are a few reasons your weight loss may have slowed down.

WEIGHT LOSS ISSUES.

Vitamin deficiency

One study showed that those who took a multivitamin lost three kilograms more a month than a control group, and that multivitamins also decreased hunger levels. Don't expect this to happen necessarily, nor to continue month after month – but there is certainly enough evidence to show that being deficient in one or more key nutrients may put the brakes on losing those last kilos.

Zinc deficiency

Zinc mimics the action of insulin, regulates inflammation and oxidative stress, and specifically helps to reduce fasting blood glucose while lowering your HbA1c level. This means zinc is a big part of blood sugar control and ultimately weight control. Consider taking around 32 milligrams daily as most people are deficient. Zinc is an important part of the digestive process, helping to produce enough stomach acid to digest food.

Selenium deficiency

Selenium is an essential micronutrient for thyroid hormone conversion and overall function. If your thyroid is sluggish, it may affect weight loss.

You may be eating too many carbs

You could still be consuming too many carbs for your metabolic rate. Unless you are actively keeping an eye on your carb count, if you are eating off the Orange list too often (or overdoing the Gold list), it's easy to overdo carbs without realising it, so it may be helpful to track your carbs for a while.

Stop all processed food

If you are not eating 100 per cent homemade-from-scratch food, you could be buying processed foods labelled as low-carb – switch to a 100 per cent wholefood diet.

Don't over-eat protein

Excess protein is converted to glucose through a process called gluconeogenesis and stored as fat. Keep a journal without being obsessive – to help you track your carbs and your protein intake. Try to aim for around one-and-a-half to two grams of protein per kilogram of bodyweight, unless you are an athlete, in which case you need more.

PROTEIN SOURCES

PROTEIN SOURCE	GRAMS OF PROTEIN	AMOUNT
Bacon	8g	6 rashers
Smoked salmon	20g	112g
Beef short ribs	24g	112g
Lamb mince	19g	112g
Pork	16g	112g
Liver pâté	16g	112g
Sardines in olive oil	12g	112g
Egg (whole egg)	7g	1
Egg yolk	3g	1
Hard cheese (Cheddar)	7g	28g
Soft cheese (Brie)	6g	28g
Sour cream, full fat	1½g	60ml

Stop fearing fat

Many people still struggle with the amount of fat, and the kind of fat, that this lifestyle requires. When you drop carbs, you need to burn something – and that something is fat. A low-carb diet coupled with low-fat is a recipe for disaster. Fat prevents hunger, improves mood and, by keeping you satisfied, prevents overeating. Healthy fat does not make you fat. Avoid seed oils and margarine, and opt instead for the healthy fats as outlined in the fats section.

Are you putting enough salt on your food?

Forget the salt myth, we all need sodium. Insulin is partly responsible for telling the kidneys not to excrete sodium, so on the LCHF diet (which brings about low insulin), you excrete more sodium; therefore, it's even more important to replenish salt or you will be short of this vital nutrient. Salt is not evil, it's an essential electrolyte.

Are you particularly carb sensitive?

It's unfair, of course it is – but some people are clearly more sensitive to carbs than others. Try going a little lower carb if you suspect you are over-sensitive, keep that food journal, work out the carb content and see whether you get a result. Cut out the unnecessary stuff and eat only real, nutritious food which nourishes the body.

Remember, this takes time

People want to lose all their weight yesterday – but the reality is that it has taken a while to pack this weight on, now you have to give it time to come off in a way that it stays off. LCHF is not a magic bullet, even though it seems to be in some fortunate people who lose huge amounts of weight with lightning speed. The reality is for most people, it's not that fast. Be realistic, this is a marathon, not a sprint. Very often people lose centimetres and have looser clothing before noticing weight loss on the scales.

No more snacking

Sorry, snacking is a death-knell if you want to lose weight – it keeps blood glucose and insulin levels high all day.

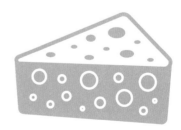

Cheating

This is merely how to sabotage yourself – just don't do it!

Sleep deprivation

There is a very strong obesity link to lack of sleep. Not getting enough sleep makes you hungrier the next day. Get a good night's sleep.

Stress

Quite bluntly, you need to manage this or it will increase cortisol, which will lead to weight gain or prevent weight loss.

Drop the artificial sweeteners

These have been shown to not only make you hungry and drive you to eat more, they actively contribute to insulin resistance.

Medication

Some medications can slow weight loss and even lead to weight gain. Don't give up, it will simply be a little slower, but you will get there. Chat to your doctor who may assist by changing your medication.

Overdoing dairy

Dairy products can spike insulin levels as much as white bread – especially in diabetics and those with insulin resistance.

Are you eating too much?

Eat your meals off a small plate and don't have seconds. Sorted.

Take supplements

Look at the supplement suggestions and try them – they may make a difference.

More things to consider

- Just because the food you eat now is healthy doesn't mean you need to eat more food. Practise restraint.
- Are you over exercising? Too much will make you hungry. Be sensible.
- If you are working out with weights you may be building muscle, which will cause the numbers on your scales to go up, but you should continue to lose centimetres.
- Do you do any exercise at all? Now might be the time to start by walking or swimming or even some high-intensity interval training (HIIT).
- Don't under-eat on carbs. If 25 grams is low, it doesn't mean five grams will be better. It's a low-carb, not a no-carb diet.
- Are you drinking too much coffee? Stimulants affect adrenal function adversely, and can sabotage weight loss.

- Do you have food sensitivities? Dairy, nuts, seeds and even eggs may be causing sensitivity. You will know this by water retention, a puffy and bloated feeling, allergies and inability to lose weight.
- Do you have a thyroid problem? Often this goes undetected or misdiagnosed, and an underactive thyroid can play havoc with your weight loss. Get medical advice.
- Are you still enjoying a glass of wine or other alcohol every night? When your body is burning alcohol, it stops burning fat. Cut all alcohol for a period of time and see if this makes a difference.
- Not eating enough vegetables – aim for at least two cups of green veggies a day.
- Eating carbs you perceive are protein (e.g. quinoa). It's classified as a grain, so leave it.
- Eating soya-based foods – never touch soya! It's toxic, fattening and damaging to the body.
- Are you eating legumes? They're unnecessary high-carb foods, plus they damage the gut. No legumes.
- Check for hidden carbs in things like sausages (often full of rusk and wheat).
- Don't make excuses for yourself when you fail; make sure you are never hungry.
- Only shop on a full stomach, never when hungry.
- Drink enough water; staying hydrated is a big secret to weight loss.

INTERMITTENT FASTING.

If you have considered all the above factors, you may want to consider what is known as intermittent fasting. This allows you to stretch the period between meals. While skipping meals may seem odd to you, it is actually far more natural than eating every few hours. For our purposes, you will start by skipping a meal, and then later maybe two – for a season.

Here are some ideas to try, as there are a few different ways that you can implement this:

1. Eat in an eight-hour window – 11am to 7pm daily. You will then be fasting for 16 hours (much of it while you are asleep, you will be relieved to know), and will eat again at 11am the next day. Drink water during this period but eat no food to spike insulin levels, and don't drink stimulants like coffee. Later you can restrict this to a five-hour window – lunch at 1pm say, and then eat again at 6pm, which gives you a longer fast period.
2. You can fast for 24 hours once a week: eat dinner on Monday night, nothing during the day on Tuesday, and then eat dinner on Tuesday evening.

While most men benefit from intermittent fasting, not all women do, and it's all to do with hormones. Please don't do this if you are pregnant, breastfeeding, diabetic (without your doctor's supervision), not getting your periods regularly, have an eating disorder of any kind, or if you have a severe illness, and please – children should not fast. If you have any doubts or problems, please speak to a health professional.

WOMEN AND WEIGHT LOSS.

There are a number of reasons why women don't have the good fortune men do when it comes to weight loss; sometimes life's just not fair.

Fat

Women have hormones! Men do too but women have more powerful ones when it comes to moods and weight loss, and we are deeply complex beings (ask any man). Our hormones particularly like storing extra padding more than men's hormones, so we have so much more to contend with.

Women tend to either eat too much fat, thinking they will lose weight the way men do on high-fat diets, or they have too little. Because women metabolise fat differently, I recommend a moderate, healthy fat intake, not a high-fat intake. Eat fat as it occurs on meat, in avocados and in nature, and dump the Bulletproof coffees.

Women are notoriously either afraid of fat, or they go overboard and drink gallons of cream and yoghurt. This is a mistake as there is no fibre present to make you feel full, and it can take a while and a lot of intoxicatingly delicious dairy before we stop and realise we have gone too far. For this reason (and others in the dairy section): ladies, leave the dairy out of your diet as far as humanly possible, except for butter.

As a woman, it is extremely important to pay attention to thyroid function. Too much caloric restriction will impact your thyroid adversely sooner or later by slowing your metabolism.

Your thyroid is too important, for both health and weight loss, to play around with. A woman is far more sensitive in terms of the thyroid gland than men are, so even going 'lower carb' should not be too low. In the last two weeks of a woman's cycle, she is less insulin sensitive than in the first two weeks. Typically though, it's in these last two weeks of the cycle that women overdo the carbs due to cravings and will experience weight gain.

Women are also notorious for giving themselves little rewards for losing a pound or two. This is called self-sabotage. We are extremely creative when it comes to excuses as to why these rewards are necessary. Enough said. Don't beat yourself up if you lose weight slowly – that's how you were designed – just keep at it and it will happen eventually for you. But don't fool yourself and don't make excuses.

05

LCHF NUTS AND BOLTS

*LCHF requires a big fridge; a medium freezer;
and a small grocery cupboard.*

– Sally-Ann Creed

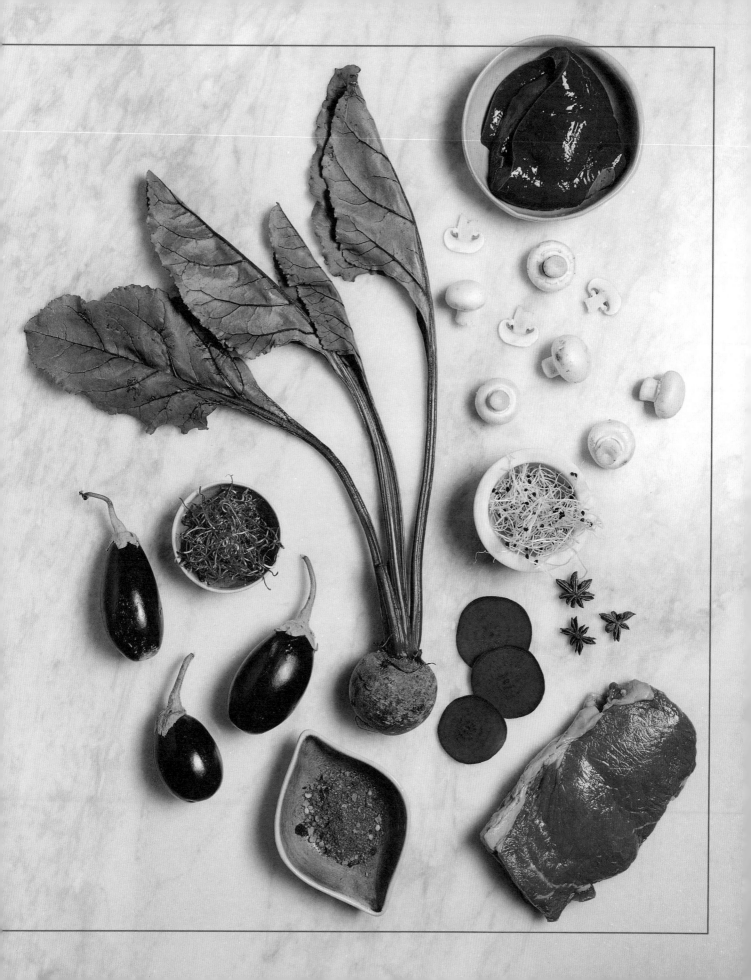

Chapter

05

SUPERFOODS

Some foods are so amazing that they help you lose weight, keep you full, heal the gut, lower inflammation in the body, boost immunity and energy levels, and literally flood your cells with nutrition.

There are some foods called 'superfoods' which are expensive, fancy-sounding foods and are often sourced from the Amazon jungle or some other exotic place on the planet. They take nine weeks of travelling by bold explorers who are at huge risk of being killed by some dangerous creature.

These are perhaps not the most natural foods to our culture after all. They cost the earth, travel vast distances, are stale when they get to you, may be poorly handled (bacteria), get irradiated on entry into the country, and half the time we don't even know what makes them so 'super' after all. If they were so super, why don't they grow here? Is it natural to eat rare foods grown at great expense to natural forestation?

There are dozens of these foods – we've all seen them. They certainly lighten the body weight fast by emptying your wallet, but that's about it.

Frankly, these are not really superfoods; they have all undergone processing of some sort or another, and are not found in their natural state.

The definition of a superfood for the purpose of this book is a wholefood as it appears in nature which has extremely high nutrient values. Let's have a look at some of nature's real superfoods, and make the most of them.

VIRGIN COCONUT OIL.

This is the most wonderfully stable oil; it won't go rancid. Coconut oil is anti-bacterial, anti-fungal and anti-ageing, while also being an amazing anti-inflammatory. It mobilises stored fat, gives endurance, is filling and really very tasty.

COCONUT MILK.

This is an athlete's dream food and an excellent alternative to dairy. Get the full-fat variety, not the reduced fat one. Coconut milk boasts saturated fatty acids and medium-chain triglycerides (MCT), which are both burned as fuel by the body and enhance athletic performance.

PASTURE-FED ANIMAL MEAT.

Whenever you can, you should try to eat pasture-fed protein, due to the higher nutrient levels, and lack of hormones and antibiotics.

Nutrients present include Vitamin E, beta-carotene, Vitamin C, and a number of health-promoting fats, including omega-3 fatty acids and conjugated linoleic acid (CLA) in pasture-fed meat, which is not present in intensively farmed meat. Did you know CLA is a powerful fat in helping you to lose weight? CLA may also be one of our most potent defences against cancer – and this is really found only in pasture-fed meat.

EGGS.

While LCHF is a moderate protein diet, we still rely heavily on protein, and eggs are an inexpensive source of superb animal protein. They are bursting with vitamins and minerals, including choline and biotin – two very important brain and liver nutrients. Eggs contain every single nutrient bar Vitamin C. They are such a perfect food you can make an entire chicken out of one! Don't be frightened of eating eggs daily if you wish. Pasture-raised eggs have 19 times higher essential fatty acid levels than ordinary supermarket eggs.

BONE BROTH.

Bone broths provide significant amounts of minerals and nutrients to our bodies, having the ability to bring about healing in a way few other foods can – this is a true super food. Nutritious juices made from boiling animal bones for an extended time, with added vegetables or herbs, and then straining out the solids, results in a broth rich in vitamins, minerals, antioxidants and amino acids. Broths are inexpensive, potent whole-body healers, which reduce inflammatory conditions, infections, boost immunity, improve bone health, heal the gut and even bring about a mood-calming effect. They strengthen your skin, hair, nails and bones.

Don't buy stocks and sauces, cubes and powders. Nothing is as powerful as the old-fashioned homemade broth. The fake alternatives you could purchase as stock are mostly chemical-based goo with hydrogenated fat and MSG, without even a passing resemblance to the real thing.

ORGAN MEATS.

This has to be one of the superstars of the meat world, as organ meats are so nutritious, and an all-time superfood group. It's hard to start eating them when you aren't used to them and find yourself over-thinking where they come from... but once you decide to take the plunge, you will realise what powerhouses of nutrition they are. Organs are the best and most nutritious part of any animal. Probably the most nutrient-dense of all, liver is the epitome of nutrition providing key nutrients like Vitamins A, D, E, K, B12 and folic acid, as well as the minerals copper and iron, helping to rid the body of ingested toxins.

BUTTER.

Everything's better with butter. It's packed with Vitamin K2, which is responsible for putting calcium in your bones and not your arteries.

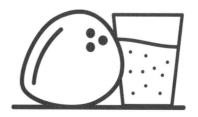

Because butter is an essential food for anyone concerned about their heart, bones, hormones and brain, it's important to mention that grass-fed butter has Vitamin K2 present – and ordinary butter from intensively farmed animals does not. Butter is also a healthy saturated fat which will raise your HDL cholesterol fraction, which is of course heart-protective.

SALMON.

The health benefits of salmon revolve around its very powerful and protective omega-3 fatty acids, EPA and DHA, which contribute to healthy brain function, heart protection, and act as very potent anti-inflammatory agents throughout the entire body.

These essential fats occur naturally in fatty fish, with the highest being found in salmon. The human body is unable to produce these vital essential fats, so they need to be eaten, and cannot be converted from other forms of omega-3 found in the plant kingdom. Not only is salmon an excellent source of high-quality protein and essential omega-3 fatty acids, it is also packed with very important vitamins and minerals such as potassium, selenium and Vitamin B12. These protect against high blood pressure, and are essential for heart health, cancer prevention and brain protection.

In the 1970s it was noted that the Inuit in Greenland ate huge amounts of fish and blubber, yet had virtually no heart disease. Scientists suggest that these essential fats protect against a variety of chronic diseases such as Alzheimer's, asthma, depression, diabetes, hypertension, macular degeneration, multiple sclerosis and rheumatoid arthritis.

FERMENTED FOODS.

Keeping our digestive systems healthy is all-important, as this is the seat of health. Fermented vegetables use beneficial bacteria that are superb at improving digestive health. Try kimchi or sauerkraut, or ferment some beets or carrots – you can Google recipes for fabulous fermented foods. If you are one of the few who can tolerate dairy, fermented dairy is an option as well. Try to aim for raw, full-fat dairy such as cultured butter if you can find it, strained yoghurt, kefir and cheeses. These healthy foods possess tremendous healing effects. Sadly, not many people tolerate dairy well, but veggies work well for most people.

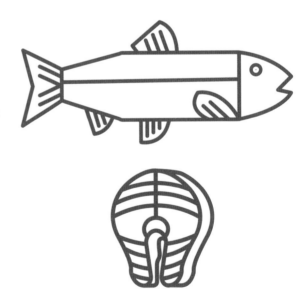

Chapter

05

SUPPLEMENTS ON LCHF

They may not be necessary if you are in peak condition, eating like a saint and feeling fantastic, but often they are an excellent adjunct to this lifestyle. This is not a definitive guide to supplementation by any stretch of the imagination, but a bird's-eye view of a few which may be helpful to you on your low-carb journey.

VITAMIN D3.

Note this is Vitamin D3 (cholecaliferol), not D2 (ergocalciferol). Some supplements merely refer to calciferol, but you need to know it is D3.

Sunshine converts cholesterol in the skin to Vitamin D; and if your cholesterol level is too low you will not be able to use the sun to generate sufficient levels of Vitamin D. If cholesterol is so dangerous, why would your body use it as precursor for Vitamin D and virtually all of the steroid hormones in your body?

Alarmingly, over 70 per cent of people are Vitamin D deficient. Perhaps get a blood test done (ask for 25(OH)) and if it's under 40,

consider upping good sources of D3 such as eggs, fatty fish and lard. The best food source of Vitamin D3 is rendered lard from pork fat; in 100 grams of lard, you get a fabulous 2,800 IU of Vitamin D3. It's vital for strong bones, uptake of calcium from food, general immune enhancement, possible better insulin sensitivity and improved weight management.

VITAMIN K2.

Vitamin K1 is primarily involved in blood clotting, while Vitamin K2 is involved in heart and bone health. It's found in grass-fed butter – the cow converts the Vitamin K1 in grass into Vitamin K2 but we cannot make that conversion. Vitamin K2 is the elusive 'factor X' discovered in healthy indigenous populations by the famous Dr Weston A Price, who studied diets around the world. He knew this substance was present in butter oil, but didn't know what the active ingredient was. In 2007, it was identified as Vitamin K2. Without it, Vitamin D will not work efficiently – both are needed to function well in the body.

In a nutshell, Vitamin K2 takes calcium and places it into the bones, not the soft tissues like the brain, cartilage or arteries where it will be troublesome. K2 builds bone in tandem with Vitamin D3. However, Vitamin K2 is thin on the ground. It's found only in a few foods in small amounts, so you could decrease your risk of osteoporosis and heart disease with a K2 supplement. Otherwise, get plenty of grass-fed butter (if the cows don't eat green grass, there's no Vitamin K1 to convert to K2), pasture-fed meats, chicken livers, hard cheeses and eggs.

MAGNESIUM.

An overlooked mineral involved in more than 300 enzymatic reactions in our bodies, magnesium is excellent for helping to normalise blood sugar levels, relax tense muscles, improve anxiety, lower hypertension, relieve constipation, prevent cramps and help you sleep like a baby. Even though it's in loads of green leafy foods, you may not get enough. If you take a supplement, magnesium citrate is a good one (not carbonate).

OMEGA-3 FISH OIL.

Omega-3 has been the darling of nutritional supplements for quite some time, as we cannot make these valuable EPA and DHA fats. We need to eat plenty of fatty fish and, if necessary, take a few grams a day of omega-3 fish oil capsules.

The benefits are huge, from dumping excess water in the body and quelling inflammation, lowering your triglyceride levels, protecting against heart disease and hardened arteries, to improving learning in children and lowering high blood pressure. You'll find the quality of your hair, skin and nails will improve, so will your memory and mood. (Flaxseed oil is not adequately converted by the body and may cause weight gain – it's not the same, so avoid this seed oil.)

L-CARNITINE.

This amino acid improves oxygen utilisation to the heart muscle, increases energy and has the added benefit of lowering triglyceride and LDL levels while raising HDL. L-Carnitine may also improve your blood sugar levels.

CHROMIUM PICOLINATE.

This is well known for increasing the rate of fat loss, lowering LDL and triglycerides while raising HDL. It facilitates the action of insulin by increasing the sensitivity of cell receptors to insulin. In other words, it makes your insulin work harder. Chromium helps curb sugar cravings and appetite in general, by up to 25 per cent, even in obese women according to a study in the journal *Diabetes Technology & Therapeutics*. Chromium appears to have the added benefit of helping to build muscle in those who work out – almost like a natural anabolic steroid.

COENZYME Q10.

If you have ever been on statins, your body will be severely depleted of this very important antioxidant. It gives the heart the ability to beat more efficiently and provides plenty of energy. It's a rejuvenating nutrient and may help significantly with weight loss, hypertension and lower LDL levels. Being cardio-protective, it is a highly recommended supplement.

VITAMIN C.

This is just such an amazing nutrient... your body cannot make it, so it's essential to eat it daily; the trouble is we cannot get enough in our food anymore. Vitamin C is a powerful antioxidant and anti-inflammatory agent, and is found in pasture-fed meats, green leafy veggies and most fresh food. It is a wonderful immune modulator, too, and is said to keep you young.

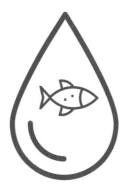

ZINC.

Zinc helps the formation of stomach acid (too little and your weight will stall) so a supplement of 32 milligrams a day is a good idea. If you are having trouble with your sense of taste and smell, have stretch marks or white marks on your nails, consider this supplement. Zinc, like chromium, helps to make your insulin more effective, thereby reducing insulin resistance.

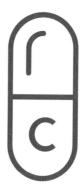

SUPPLEMENT SUMMARY

Dosages are for adults who weigh more than 8 stone (50kg). As with everything else in this book, if there is any doubt, please speak to your qualified healthcare provider first.

Vitamin D3	2,000-10,000 iu/day depending on blood results	**Co-Q10**	60mg-120mg/day
Vitamin K2	180-200mcg/day of MK-7 and MK-4 (mixed)	**Vitamin C**	Anything from 500mg to as high as you would like to go – 2g is okay
Fish oil	1-3g is usually adequate	**Chromium**	1 to 6 x 200mcg capsules a day in divided doses (1-2, 3 x a day)
Magnesium	400-600mg a day (magnesium citrate or glycinate is recommended)	**Zinc**	22-50mg a day
		Probiotics	The best you can lay your hands on with a high CFU count
L-Carnitine	500mg-2g/day		

Chapter

05

PREBIOTICS AND PROBIOTICS

"All disease begins in the gut", to quote Hippocrates, the father of medicine. In order to understand the difference between pre- and probiotics, let's clarify it this way: prebiotics are indigestible carbohydrates which are food for probiotics. Probiotics are beneficial organisms living in the digestive tract. We recommend eating prebiotic foods like kefir, sauerkraut and kimchi plus organic apple cider vinegar and bone broth – all of which enable you to increase healthy gut flora. Get a good probiotic from a qualified nutritional therapist, as we are usually woefully short of healthy gut flora. Eating a real food diet devoid of junk food is the first step to a healthy digestive system.

Did you know that you are 10 per cent human and 90 per cent bacteria? In terms of genes, only 10 per cent of our genes dictate who we are, according to the Human Microbiome Project. There are more than 10,000 microbial species we cart around with us, and they contribute more genes responsible for our survival than those we are born with. We cannot live without this wonderful microbiome inside us. Together with our own genes, they make up who we are. We should be ever-mindful of the importance our gut plays in weight loss, health and even how we think and feel. Gut health dictates our immunity, sleep, moods and whether or not we contract certain diseases or side-step them.

THE BENEFITS OF GUT HEALTH.

By strengthening your digestive system and at the same time improving your entire gut ecology, you will find many underlying health conditions may clear up, and quite quickly too – including a possible stubborn inability to shed unwanted extra weight. There is no magic bullet here, but probiotics have been shown to help with the following conditions:

- Antibiotic-induced diarrhoea
- Urinary tract infections
- Vaginal yeast infections, such as candida strains
- Eczema and many other skin complaints
- Food allergies/intolerances
- Cancer
- Irritable bowel syndrome
- Inflammatory bowel disease
- Ulcerative colitis
- Crohn's disease
- Traveller's diarrhoea
- Improved digestion and bowel movements

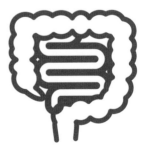

GUT INSTINCT.

Results all depend on whether the supplement has real, live bacteria present, how strong it is and whether it's actually able to make an impression. You could equate the strains to varieties of fuchsia plants. You have many varieties and colours – purple, white, red – they are all fuchsias, yet they vary in shape, size, hardiness and appearance. In a similar fashion, the varied strains of gut bacteria have multiple functions and characteristics; whereas some are very strong and hardy, others are weak, fragile and sensitive.

Probiotics also have very specific jobs they need to do; one important task is preventing urinary tract infections (UTI). The bacteria present in the vagina and urethra are made up primarily by lactobacilli, which act as a barrier to UTIs. These also prevent antibiotic-induced diarrhoea, a common antibiotic problem.

Incidentally, it's not true that you should wait until you've finished your course of antibiotics before taking probiotics – the research strongly supports that you take them while on antibiotics; just make sure to take them around three to four hours away from antibiotics.

GUT FEELING

You could say that prebiotics are fertilisers which encourage healthy bacterial growth, as they feed them and promote their proliferation. Some foods which encourage healthy bacteria include:

Tomatoes	Kefir
Artichokes	Buttermilk
Onions	Aged cheeses
Garlic	Olives
Chicory	Beans
Dandelion greens	Kombucha
Asparagus	Fermented vegetables
Leeks	Sauerkraut
Berries	Kimchi
Green bananas	Brined pickles
Yoghurt	

SUPPLEMENTS WHICH ENCOURAGE HEALTHY BACTERIA

- L-Glutamine
- Zinc
- Vitamin A (you can get this from liver)
- Probiotics (there are various brands – so get a good one)

TYPES OF BACTERIA

GOOD BACTERIA	BAD BACTERIA
Bifidobacteria – These strains regulate all the levels of the other bacteria in the gut as well as modulating immune responses to invading pathogens. They prevent tumour formation and even produce some vitamins and short-chain fatty acids.	**Campylobacter** – C.jejuni and C.coli are the most common strains associated with humans. Usually this is picked up from contaminated food.
Escherichia coli – There are many different types present in the human digestive tract, and these are involved in the production of Vitamin K2, plus they help to keep bad bacteria under control; some strains do lead to illness though.	**Enterococcus faecalis** – A very common cause of post-surgical infection.
Lactobacilli – There are many beneficial varieties of this organism which manufacture nutrients. They help to boost immunity and protect against cancer-causing agents.	**Clostridium difficile** – This is possibly the most harmful one and often occurs after a course or several courses of antibiotics – the best time for it to multiply.

There can be hundreds of strains of probiotic flora present in the human gut, these are just a few to show you what some of the more common ones do, and the importance of the gut in the whole health scenario. It's ideal to have the full complement of beneficial strains, and caring for your gut will make sure you have the best chance.

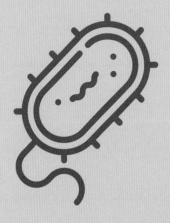

Chapter

05

TROUBLESHOOTING

People on a LCHF diet often have a few problems when they transition from a low-fat high-carb diet to the exact opposite. Here are a few common problems you may face.

LCHF WITHOUT A GALLBLADDER.

This is absolutely fine. The gallbladder is simply responsible for storing bile produced by the liver. Bile is used to aid in the digestion of dietary fats – the liver still continues to make it even without the little storage organ – the gallbladder. Simply introduce it slowly and spread your fat intake out throughout the day to enable the body to get used to eating fat again. Bile empties directly into the small intestine as an emulsifier for fats, much like dishwashing liquid breaks up fats from the saucepan in hot soapy water, turning it into a slurry for digestion.

CRAMPS.

Cramps can happen to people whether they are following a low-carb lifestyle or not. However, it's a common symptom when you begin LCHF. By limiting carbohydrates, your body retains less water and rids itself of water via the kidneys, taking a lot of stored magnesium and salt with it.

Remain adequately hydrated by drinking plenty of water and make sure you have enough salt in your food (add extra to water if you need to), and take a magnesium citrate supplement. Insulin signals the kidneys to retain salt so low insulin allows salt excretion, which can lead to cramps. Bone broth is another amazing way to deal with cramps.

CONSTIPATION.

Remaining adequately hydrated with water should help enormously. Magnesium, fibre from your food and perhaps adding in a fibre supplement like chia seeds or psyllium husks will help. Whenever any dietary change is made, the body will have to undergo adjustments, and constipation is usually quite normal during this time. More salt and magnesium is the first place to start, and do some stretches before bed.

LOW-CARB OR KETO 'FLU'.

This isn't really a flu, you are just going through a withdrawal from the toxic foods you have now discontinued. It could last anywhere from a day to two weeks, and be mild or severe – or you may not experience anything. Try to remind yourself that you are ridding your body of toxins from all the abuse it's had from high-carbohydrate diets and junk food – it gets worse before it gets better. You could try a few of the following methods to alleviate the discomfort:

- Drink plenty of water
- Increase your salt and magnesium intake
- Drink chicken or bone broth (homemade) throughout the day
- Take 1 gram of Vitamin C every few hours
- Take a Vitamin B6 if you are very moody (use the P-5-P kind, a bioavailable form)
- Take omega-3 fish oils – around three grams a day

BAD BREATH.

As you become fat adapted, your body will produce ketones which can be smelled in your sweat, urine or breath. The smell of acetone on the breath is akin to nail polish remover or ammonia, but don't worry, it won't last long and will be gone in a few days if you keep hydrated and have plenty of deodorising leafy greens. Make sure that you are having moderate protein intake, and enough leafy greens.

INSOMNIA.

This is a common effect whenever you radically change your diet. The body will have to adjust to new foods, new nutrient levels, hydration levels and various other pattern changes. This can be stressful to the body, so cortisol tends to increase when you embark on a new dietary regimen, which can affect sleep patterns at first – this quickly changes though, and you should be sleeping like a baby in no time. Try a bath in a weak solution of Epsom salts before bed – this helps a lot too.

DIZZINESS.

Blood pressure can drop quite quickly once all those carbs and sugars are removed from the diet. Other reasons could be too little salt or magnesium. If you are on blood pressure medication, have your blood pressure and medication monitored by your GP or healthcare provider regularly especially in the first few weeks. It may have become too strong or you could be suffering from low blood pressure.

HEART PALPITATIONS.

It is common to experience faster or stronger heart beats during the first few weeks, and while it's uncomfortable, it's generally nothing to worry about. More water, a little more salt and magnesium usually sorts this out.

If this doesn't eliminate the symptom completely, perhaps you are too stressed – managing stress is extremely important. Don't underestimate the initial stress that a change in dietary habits puts on the body (in this case it's good, but it's a stressor nonetheless).

FATIGUE.

You may experience fatigue in the first week or so – also very normal. If it continues though, it's possible you are not eating enough fat or protein. So make sure you are getting enough healthy fat, protein and green leafy veggies. And make sure all the sugar is out of your diet.

TEMPORARY HAIR LOSS.

Hair loss occurs for many reasons including illness, stress, pregnancy, breastfeeding, starvation and low levels of protein. Regarding the change of diet, the hair loss may occur usually three to six months into your new lifestyle; it is temporary and will soon normalise.

Everyone's hair goes into a 'resting phase' every now and then, but we seem to notice it more when we change from one diet to another as there is additional hair loss during this time. It will rectify itself – give it time, and make sure you have enough protein and fat, and that you are not anaemic.

PERIOD CHANGES.

You may find your period changes to become more regular or goes away for a season. If the latter, make sure you are eating enough fat. Remember, very often this way of life makes you more fertile.

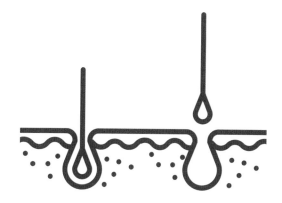

A WEEK'S LCHF MENU

	MONDAY	TUESDAY	WEDNESDAY	THURSDAY	FRIDAY	SATURDAY	SUNDAY
BREAKFAST	2-3 egg omelette in butter, wilted spinach and lightly sautéed cherry tomatoes	Beef liver or chicken livers with asparagus or green beans and a little fried onion	Egg Muffins (p160) with bacon, mushroom and cheese	Smoked salmon on a bed of **rocket or lettuce leaves**, ½ avocado, salt and pepper and a drizzle of olive oil	Fried egg with a small healthy sausage and six steamed asparagus spears with melted butter, salt and pepper	Bacon and Spinach Frittata (p165)	Poached or scrambled eggs on 2 rounds of sautéed, aubergine, rocket and asparagus, top with bacon
LUNCH	120g diced chicken and skin with Homemade Mayonnaise (p216) or Creamy Salad Dressing (p214) with leafy salad greens from the Green list (cos lettuce, rocket, tomatoes, cucumber)	Tuna salad (tinned in brine): tuna, tomato, cucumber, little onion, red peppers, coriander, Homemade Mayonnaise served on shredded lettuce	Tin of sardines (in brine or olive oil) on a Olive and Rosemary Seed Cracker (p220) with butter. Add Sweet Red Pepper Chilli **Relish (p218)** and lettuce, rocket and avocado	Chicken Liver **Salad (p178)**	Des's Curry served on sautéed cabbage ribbons or cauli-rice or broccoli rice (brolli-rice)	Baked hake in the oven with butter, lemon wedges, salt and pepper with a Green list salad, olive oil and apple cider vinegar, few seeds and nuts sprinkled over the top	Pumpkin Soup (p206), 1 slice Courgette Bread (p222) Or in summer, 2-3 grilled lamb chops on cauli-mash with gem squash, broccoli and dripping made into a 'gravy'
DINNER	2-3 grilled or roasted lamb chops with cauli-mash and broccoli. Side of your choice (p192)	Zoodles and Meatballs (p169)	Roast chicken leg and thigh, baby marrows, ½ gem squash done in the oven with a little blue cheese, red bell peppers sautéed with mushrooms in butter – pour sauce over the chicken	Curry (p166) with cauli-rice, cabbage strips or zucchini noodles. Small side salsa of chopped tomato and ¼ thinly sliced and chopped onion if you wish	Roast belly of pork, Broccoli with Mustard **Butter (p194)** gem squash with butter, asparagus lightly boiled and drizzled with butter or Liquidiser Hollandaise (p214), well seasoned and sprinkled with almond flakes or pine nuts	Barbecue night: any choice of meat with Tabouli (p210), Coleslaw (p198) Pudding: Baked Vanilla Custard (p236)	Bunless burger on large mushrooms (sautéed/roasted) with grated cheese, tomato slice, lettuce and Sweet Red Pepper Chilli Relish and/or Homemade Mayonnaise
TREATS	125ml Greek yoghurt	Cream in coffee	Hot/iced cocoa	Chia 'porridge'	Applesauce (pork)		

Beverages suggested

- Black coffee (MSG-free)
- Coffee (whole milk or cream)
- Tea (any leaf teas)
- Water
- Bone broth

KIDS (extras if needed)

Add in foods from Orange list
1 fruit a day (pref. not grapes)
Low-carb homemade muffin
Yoghurt, extra cheese, few nuts
Any Orange list vegetables

Snacks (if necessary)

- Biltong (MSG-free)
- Activated nuts
- Low-carb muffin (small)
- Nuts, cheese
- Boiled egg (snacks don't have to be sweet or bready)

A WEEK'S AFFORDABLE MENU WHICH WON'T BREAK THE BANK

	MONDAY	TUESDAY	WEDNESDAY	THURSDAY	FRIDAY	SATURDAY	SUNDAY
BREAKFAST	Scrambled eggs in butter or rendered pork fat on a bed of spinach, cabbage or any Green list vegetable	Omelette with any Green list veg from last night (lovely re-heated) or flat sautéed courgette ribbons	Bacon and Spinach Fritatta variation (p165)	Aubergine Stack topped with a fried egg, basil leaves and rocket/lettuce (p162)	Boiled eggs with Olive and Rosemary Seed Crackers and butter, topped with thinly sliced tomato and seasoned well	Fried egg with leftover mince on wilted spinach	Fried Brawn (p172) with tomato and a little onion (the brawn will melt in the pan), topped with scrambled or poached egg
LUNCH	Chicken Broth (p208) with Olive and Rosemary Seed Crackers and butter; or if it's summer, Coronation Chicken (p184) with avocado and tomato	Leftover Fish Pie from last night with a crispy salad, ½ avocado, drizzled olive oil and apple cider vinegar	Cheesy Portobello Mushrooms (p177), with lettuce, tomato and cucumber ribbons	Leftover Pork Trotters and cabbage (it's nicer than you think)	Tin of sardines or tuna (in brine or olive oil) on a Olive and Rosemary Seed Cracker with butter. Add Versatile Tomato Sauce (p217) and lettuce, rocket and avocado	Baked or fried hake with lemon butter, garden herbs and a crisp green salad with olive oil and apple cider vinegar	Leftover Coconut Thai Green Chicken Curry. Have a little mashed sweet potato or pumpkin as a treat
DINNER	Fish Pie (p170) with seasonal Green list veggies, stir-fried in lard (spinach, cabbage, cauliflower, broccoli)	Chicken livers with stir-fried veggies (cabbage, spinach, peppers, little onion, mushrooms)	Pork Trotters (p175) on braised and seasoned cabbage	Chicken and vegetable soup; if summer, Cabbage Carbonara (p187)	Fatty minced pork/lamb/beef sautéed with a little garlic and onion, seasoning and simmered, served on a bed of cabbage strips steamed and then buttered with salt and cracked black pepper	Coconut Thai Green Chicken Curry (p181) with cauli-rice or salad greens	Chicken breast burgers without buns – serve breast between two thick slices of sautéed aubergine, with lettuce, tomato and a slice of onion. Add Homemade Mayonnaise and Sweet Red Pepper Chilli Relish
ADDITIONS FOR KIDS	Small sweet potato/pumpkin	Piece of fruit (apple, pear, tart fruit)	Add some grated raw beetroot and/ or carrot to the salad	Braised carrots can be added to a meal, or grated over a salad	Baby turnips mashed with butter and cream cheese	Greek yoghurt with berries and a few nuts	Coffee with cream and no sugar; home-flavoured waters

For an affordable menu, I feel a dessert is not necessary. Desserts are by nature expensive. However, if you want to whip one up, you'll get the most bang for your buck with the Light and Fluffy Chocolate Mousse on page 241.

Chapter

05

THE OFFICIAL UPDATED LISTS

The lists have had to be updated from the original red book lists due to the changing landscape of LCHF. In an attempt to help clear up the confusion, there are four main lists with a banned list at the end. The Green and Red lists have been simplified and divided to more accurately depict food values.

NOTES.

- All amounts on these lists are net carbs, raw weight, and depict carbs per 100g.
- Some foods have been moved to adhere strictly to the net carb grams per 100 grams rule (e.g. balsamic vinegar at 3g per tablespoon is okay, but over 100g would significantly overshoot the less than 5g/100 rule for Green or Gold listing). The same applies for spices such as garlic and black pepper on the Red list.
- Banned foods are unhealthy and should be avoided, no matter what the carb count is.

GUIDE TO THE NEW LISTS.

GREEN LIST
Eat freely: 0-5g/100g net carbs.

GOLD LIST
Mainly protein and fat. Energy-dense foods. Carbs = 0-5g/100. Exercise portion control, excess may prevent weight loss. Eat dairy frugally as it is insulinogenic and obesogenic.

ORANGE LIST
Wholefoods from 5.1-25g/100g to be counted into daily carb 'budget'. Higher carb foods, may suit a Paleo/Primal approach to LCHF.

RED LIST
High-carb foods >25.1g/100g. Mostly wholefoods may not be suitable for LCHF or weight loss. Paleo enthusiasts may still wish to use some of these foods.

BANNED LIST
Substances regarded as either harmful to the body, are damaged due to processing, synthetic, not wholefoods, or may present health problems. Carb counts are irrelevant – it's a never-ever list.

These new lists supersede the old lists – they are fully updated, and these may now be used as updated Real Food Low-Carb lists. Stick mainly to the Green and Gold lists (0-5/100g), with some restraint needed from the Gold list. The new colour coding will help you to not overeat without realising it. Eat from the Green and Gold lists daily – choose more sensibly from the Gold list.

SUMMARY.

Green: Eat all you like <5g/100g
Gold: Eat in moderation <5/100g
                (energy dense)
Orange: Wholefoods 5.1g-25g/100g
                (higher in carbs)
Red: Wholefoods >25.1g/100
                (high-carb foods)
Banned: Unhealthy, harmful, processed
                – forget the carbs, these are out!

NOTES.

Food in its raw state is very different in nutritional value to its fermented, cooked, baked, boiled, stewed or fried state. There are also many different varieties of the same food. For example: 100g of potatoes with skin and flesh raw is approximately 15.39g net carbs (and this is just one variety of potato), but when you bake this same potato with skin and flesh together, the net carbs increase to 18.95g; microwave the same potato and the net carbs soar to 21.94g carbs. (Of course, we know you won't do anything as unhealthy as microwaving, will you?). This holds true for most foods.

Food in different forms and under different circumstances changes some of the values of that food slightly. The length of time fruit is left to ripen on the tree, how long it's kept in the fridge, how it's packaged, where it is farmed; these all change its nutritional value. We can only give estimates according to data put out by the USDA and other reliable institutions.

The lists are created based on raw nutritional information and cannot ever be 100 per cent accurate because no two apples have exactly the same nutritional value. We could not possibly provide a list of foods for every conceivable variety of squash or every type of cooked or raw vegetable either. We have elected to categorise foods in their raw state, as this is more consistent than using their cooked or baked weight, and include only the most common foods. Obscure foods take up space and become overwhelming – there are online sources for these.

The following tables outline the Green, Gold, Orange, Red and Banned lists. Please note, wherever you see "-" no data was available at the time of going to print.

THE GREEN LIST

GREEN: 0-5G NET CARBS PER 100G (EAT FREELY) FRUIT AND VEGETABLES	CALORIES	PROTEIN	TOTAL FAT	CARBS	FIBRE	NET CARBS	SUGAR
Alfalfa sprouts	23	3,99	0,69	2,1	1,9	0,2	0,2
Asparagus	20	2,2	0,12	3,88	2,1	1,78	1,88
Aubergine (eggplant)	25	0,98	0,18	5,88	3	2,88	3,53
Avocado	160	2	14,66	8,53	6,7	1,83	0,66
Bamboo shoots	27	2,6	0,3	5,2	2,2	3	3
Basil	23	3,15	0,64	2,65	1,6	1,05	0,3
Bean sprouts, mung beans	30	3,04	0,18	5,94	1,8	4,14	4,13
Beans, green, snap	31	1,83	0,22	6,97	2,7	4,27	3,26
Beet greens	22	2,2	0,13	4,33	3,7	0,63	0,5
Blackberries	43	1,39	0,49	9,61	5,3	4,31	4,88
Broccoli	34	2,82	0,37	6,64	2,6	4,04	1,7
Cabbage, white	24	1,21	0,18	5,37	2,3	3,07	3
Cauliflower	25	1,92	0,28	4,97	2	2,97	1,91
Celery	16	0,69	0,17	2,97	1,6	1,37	1,34
Chard	19	1,8	0,2	3,74	1,6	2,14	1,1
Chicory greens	23	1,7	0,3	4,7	4	0,7	0,7
Chives	30	3,27	0,73	4,35	2,5	1,85	1,85
Cress, garden	32	2,6	0,7	5,5	1,1	4,4	4,4
Cucumber with skin	15	0,65	0,11	3,63	0,5	3,13	1,67
Dill	43	3,46	1,12	7,02	2,1	4,92	0
Dill pickles (note: pickle juice can contain sugar), cucumber, dill	12	0,5	0,3	2,41	1	1,41	1,07
Endive	17	1,25	0,2	3,35	3,1	0,25	0,25
Fennel bulb	31	1,24	0,2	7,3	3,1	4,2	3,93
Gem squash	15,97	2,9	1,5	3,4	1,1	2,3	1,7
Kimchi, cabbage	15	1,1	0,5	2,4	1,6	0,8	1,06
Kohlrabi	27	1,7	0,1	6,2	3,6	2,6	2,6
Lettuce	15	1,36	0,15	2,87	1,3	1,57	0,78
Mangetout (flat pod, no peas inside)	38	4	0	4	2	2	2
Mushrooms, maitake	31	1,94	0,19	6,97	2,7	4,27	2,07
Mushrooms, oyster	33	3,31	0,41	6,09	2,3	3,79	1,11
Mushrooms, white	22	3,09	0,34	3,26	1	2,26	1,98
Mustard greens	27	2,86	0,42	4,67	3,2	1,47	1,32
Okra	33	1,93	0,19	7,45	3,2	4,25	1,48
Olives, green	145	1,03	15,32	3,84	3,3	0,54	0,54
Parsley	36	2,97	0,79	6,33	3,3	3,03	0,85
Pattypans	18	1,2	0,2	3,84	1,2	2,64	2,39
Peppers, green	20	0,86	1,7	4,64	1,7	2,94	2,4
Peppers, red	31	0,99	0,3	6,03	2,1	3,93	4,2
Pok choi	13	1,5	0,2	2,18	1	1,18	1,18

THE GREEN LIST

GREEN: 0-5G NET CARBS PER 100G (EAT FREELY)	CALORIES	PROTEIN	TOTAL FAT	CARBS	FIBRE	NET CARBS	SUGAR
Radicchio	23	1,43	0,25	4,48	0,9	3,58	0,6
Radish	16	0,68	0,1	3,4	1,6	1,8	1,86
Rhubarb	21	0,9	0,2	4,54	1,8	2,74	1,1
Rocket (arugula)	25	2,58	0,66	3,65	1,6	2,05	2,05
Sauerkraut	90	0,91	0,14	4,28	2,9	1,38	1,78
Scallions, spring onions	32	1,83	0,19	7,34	2,6	4,74	2,33
Seaweed	26	5,92	0,39	2,42	0,4	2,02	0,3
Spearmint, fresh	44	3,29	0,73	8,41	6,8	1,61	-
Spinach	23	2,86	0,39	3,63	2,2	1,43	0,42
Sprouts, alfalfa	23	3,99	0,69	2,1	1,9	0,2	0,2
Starfruit	31	1,04	0,33	6,73	2,8	3,93	3,98
Swiss chard	19	1,8	0,2	3,74	1,6	2,14	1,1
Tomatillos	32	0,96	1,02	5,84	1,9	3,94	3,93
Tomatoes	18	0,88	0,2	3,89	1,2	2,69	2,63
Turnips	28	0,9	0,1	6,43	1,8	4,63	3,8
Waterblommetjies	38	1	0	4	5	0	3
Watercress	11	2,3	0,1	1,29	0,5	0,79	0,2
Zucchini	21	2,71	0,4	3,11	1,1	2,01	-
SWEETENERS							
Erythritol granules	0	0	0	0	0	0	0
Stevia powder	0	0	0	0	0	0	0
Xylitol granules	0	0	0	0	0	0	0
BEVERAGES							
Coconut water from fresh green coconuts	19	0,72	0,2	3,71	1,1	2,61	2,61
Fruit-infused waters (homemade only)	0	0	0	0	0	0	-
Rooibos tea	0	0	0	0	0	0	0
Sparkling water	0	0	0	0	0	0	0
Spring water	0	0	0	0	0	0	0
Tea, black	1	0	0	0,2	0	0,2	0
Whole leaf herbal teas with no additives	0	0	0	0	0	0	-
CONDIMENTS, HERBS AND SPICES							
Cider vinegar	21	0	0	0,93	0	0,93	0,4
Curry powder (preferably homemade)	325	14,29	14,01	55,83	53,2	2,63	2,76
Gelatine	335	85,6	0,1	0	0	0	0
Mustard, Dijon	66	3,95	3,11	7,78	3,2	4,58	2,84
Red wine vinegar	19	0,04	0	0,27	0	0,27	0
Rock salt	0	0	0	0	0	0	0
Tabasco sauce	12	1,29	0,76	0,8	0,6	0,2	0,13
Vinegars, distilled	18	0	0	0,04	0	0,04	0,04
OTHER							
Psyllium husk powder	357	0	0	100	100	0	0
Xanthan gum	292	0	0	67	67	0	0

THE GOLD LIST

GOLD: 0-5G NET CARBS PER 100G (BUT NOT AN ALL-YOU-CAN-EAT LIST) MEAT	CALORIES	PROTEIN	TOTAL FAT	CARBS	FIBRE	NET CARBS	SUGAR
All animal meats are allowed. Must be free from marinades, preferably hormone-free and humanely reared.							
Antelope	114	22,38	2,03	0	0	0	0
Bacon	417	12,62	39,69	1,28	0	1,28	1
Beef, ground, 80% lean meat, 20% fat, raw	254	17,17	20	0	0	0	0
Biltong	250	51,99	5	0,23	0	0,23	0
Blood sausage/black pudding	379	14,6	34,5	1,29	0	1,29	0
Bockwurst, pork veal	301	14,03	25,87	2,95	1	1,95	1,33
Brains, beef and by-products	143	10,86	10,3	1,05	0	1,05	0
Brains, lamb and by-products	122	10,4	8,58	0	0	0	0
Brains, pork and by-products	127	10,28	9,21	0	0	0	0
Chicken broilers, meat and skin	215	18,6	15,06	0	0	0	0
Chicken eggs, raw	143	12,56	9,51	0,72	0	0,72	0,37
Chicken giblets	124	17,88	4,47	1,8	0	1,8	0
Chicken gizzards	94	17,66	2,06	0	0	0	0
Chicken hearts, raw	153	15,55	9,33	0,71	0	0,71	0
Chicken livers	119	16,92	4,83	0,73	0	0,73	0
Chorizo, pork and beef	455	24,1	38,27	1,86	0	1,86	0
Cornish hen, meat and skin	200	17,15	14,02	0	0	0	0
Deer	120	22,96	2,42	0	0	0	0
Duck eggs	185	12,81	13,77	1,45	0	1,45	0
Duck liver	136	18,74	4,64	3,53	0	3,53	0
Duck, wild, meat and skin	211	17,42	15,2	0	0	0	0
Elk	111	22,95	1,45	0	0	0	0
Emu	134	22,77	4,03	0	0	0	0
Gelatines, unsweetened, dry powder	335	85,6	0,1	0	0	0	0
Goat	109	20,6	2,31	0	0	0	0
Goose egg	185	13,87	13,27	1,35	0	1,35	0
Goose, meat and skin	371	15,86	33,62	0	0	0	0
Guinea fowl, meat and skin	158	23,4	6,45	0	0	0	0
Kidney, beef	99	17,4	3,09	0,29	0	0,29	0
Kidney, lamb	97	15,74	2,95	0,82	0	0,82	0
Kidney, pork	100	16,46	3,25	0	0	0	0
Lamb quarters	43	4,2	0,8	7,3	4	3,3	0
Lamb mince	282	16,56	23,41	0	0	0	0
Liver, beef	135	20,36	3,63	3,89	0	3,89	0
Liver, lamb	139	20,38	5,02	1,78	0	1,78	0
Liver, veal	140	19,93	4,85	2,91	0	2,91	0
Ostrich (iffy due to hormones used – check source)	165	20,22	8,7	0	0	0	0
Pastrami, beef	147	21,8	5,82	0,36	0	0,36	0,1
Pigeon/squab, meat and skin	294	18,47	23,8	0	0	0	0

THE GOLD LIST

MEAT	CALORIES	PROTEIN	TOTAL FAT	CARBS	FIBRE	NET CARBS	SUGAR
Pork belly	518	9,34	53,01	0	0	0	0
Pork meat	211	18,22	14,79	0	0	0	0
Quail eggs	158	13,05	11,09	0,41	0	0,41	0
Quail, meat and skin	192	19,63	12,05	0	0	0	0
Rabbit	114	21,79	2,32	0	0	0	0
Salami, pork	425	21,7	37	1,2	0	1,2	0
Sausage, Italian, pork (avoid those with gluten, MSG and additives)	346	14,25	31,33	0,65	0	0,65	0
Snail	90	16,1	1,4	2	0	2	0
Turkey egg	171	13,68	11,88	1,15	0	1,15	0
Turkey, whole, meat and skin	143	21,64	5,64	0,13	0	0,13	0
Veal (preferably not though, due to the cruelty in rearing veal)	197	18,58	13,06	0	0	0	0
Venison	116	21,05	2,66	0	0	0	0
SEAFOOD							
Fish – all (except swordfish and tilefish due to high mercury)							
Canned seafood – check labels for added carbs. Best in brine or olive oil.							
Anchovies	131	20,35	4,84	0	0	0	0
Barbel	95	16,38	2,82	0	0	0	0
Butterfish	146	17,28	8,02	0	0	0	0
Carp	127	17,83	5,6	0	0	0	0
Caviar, black/red granular	264	24,6	17,9	4	0	4	0
Couta	105	20,28	2	0	0	0	0
Crustaceans – all (lobster, clams, crabs, crayfish, scallops, mussels)	71	13,61	1,01	0,91	0	0,91	0
Eel	184	18,44	11,66	0	0	0	0
Fish broth	16	2	0,6	0,4	0	0,4	0,09
Haddock	74	16,32	0,45	0	0	0	0
Herring, Atlantic	158	17,96	9,04	0	0	0	0
Kingklip	77	17,2	0,4	0	0	0	0
Mackerel, Atlantic	205	18,6	13,89	0	0	0	0
Monkfish	76	14,48	1,52	0	0	0	0
Mullet	117	19,35	3,79	0	0	0	0
Octopus	82	14,9	1,04	2,2	0	2,2	0
Oyster, Pacific	81	9,45	2,3	4,95	0	4,95	0
Rock cod	92	19,38	1,02	0	0	0	0
Salmon, Atlantic	142	19,84	6,34	0	0	0	0
Salmon, pink	127	20,5	4,4	0	0	0	0
Sardines, tinned and drained, with bones	208	24,62	11,45	0	0	0	0
Sea bass	97	18,43	2	0	0	0	0
Shad	197	16,93	13,77	0	0	0	0
Shrimp, canned	100	20,42	1,36	0	0	0	0
Snapper	100	20,51	1,34	0	0	0	0
Sole	70	12,41	1,93	0	0	0	0

THE GOLD LIST

SEAFOOD	CALORIES	PROTEIN	TOTAL FAT	CARBS	FIBRE	NET CARBS	SUGAR
Squid/calamari	92	15,58	1,38	3,08	0	3,08	0
Trout, mixed species	148	20,77	6,61	0	0	0	0
Tuna, yellowfin, fresh	144	23,3	4,9	0	0	0	0
Yellowtail	146	23,14	5,24	0	0	0	0
FATS							
Butter, salted or unsalted	717	0,85	81,11	0,06	0	0	0,06
Chicken fat	900	0	99,8	0	0	0	0
Cocoa butter	884	0	100	0	0	0	0
Coconut oil	892	0	99,06	0	0	0	0
Duck fat	882	0	99,8	0	0	0	0
Goose fat	900	0	99,8	0	0	0	0
Lard (pork not vegetable lard)	902	0	100	0	0	0	0
Medium-chain triglyceride oil (MCT oil)	839	0	92,4	0	0	0	0
Oil, avocado	884	0	100	0	0	0	0
Oil, hazelnut	884	0	100	0	0	0	0
Oil, macadamia	796	0	90.4	0	0	0	0
Oil, palm (organic, red palm oil – not hydrogenated)	884	0	100	0	0	0	0
Oil, walnut	884	0	100	0	0	0	0
Olive oil (extra virgin only – and always in glass)	119	0	13,5	0	0	0	0
Olives, canned or pickled	145	1,03	15,32	3,84	3,3	0,54	0,54
Tallow, beef	902	0	100	0	0	0	0
Tallow, lamb, mutton	902	0	100	0	0	0	0
Turkey fat	900	0	99,8	0	0	0	0
DAIRY AND RELATED							
Blue cheese	353	21,4	28,74	2,34	0	2,34	0,5
Brie cheese	334	20,75	27,68	0,45	0	0,45	0,45
Buttermilk, whole	62	3,21	3,31	4,88	0	4,88	4,88
Camembert	300	19,8	24,26	0,46	0	0,46	0,46
Cheddar cheese	404	22,87	33,31	3,09	0	3,09	0,48
Coconut cream (unsweetened)	330	3,63	34,68	6,65	2,2	4,45	-
Coconut milk (unsweetened)	230	2,29	23,84	5,54	2,2	3,34	3,34
Cottage cheese, full fat	98	11,12	4,3	3,38	0	3,38	2,67
Cream, double, fresh	340	2,84	36,08	2,74	0	2,74	2,92
Cream, single, fresh	191	2,96	19,1	2,82	0	2,82	3,67
Cream, sour	198	2,44	19,35	4,63	0	4,63	3,41
Edam cheese	357	24,99	27,8	1,43	0	1,43	1,43
Feta cheese	264	14,21	21,28	4,09	0	4,09	4,09
Fontina cheese	389	25,6	31,14	1,55	0	1,55	1,55
Goat's cheese, hard	452	30,52	35,59	2,17	0	2,17	2,17
Goat's cheese, soft	264	18,52	21,08	0	0	0	0
Goat's milk	69	3,56	4,14	4,45	0	4,45	4,45

THE GOLD LIST

DAIRY AND RELATED	CALORIES	PROTEIN	TOTAL FAT	CARBS	FIBRE	NET CARBS	SUGAR
Gouda cheese	356	24,94	27,44	2,22	0	2,22	2,22
Gruyere cheese	413	29,81	32,34	0,36	0	0,36	0,36
Limburger cheese	327	20,05	27,25	0,49	0	0,49	0,49
Milk, whole	61	3,15	3,27	4,78	0	4,78	4,78
Monterey cheese	373	24,48	30,28	0,68	0	0,68	0,5
Mozzarella	300	22,17	22,35	2,19	0	2,19	1,03
Parmesan cheese, hard	392	35,75	25,83	3,22	0	3,22	0,8
Ricotta cheese	174	11,26	12,98	3,04	0	3,04	0,27
Romano cheese	387	31,8	26,94	3,63	0	3,63	0,73
Roquefort cheese	369	21,54	30,64	2	0	2	0
Swiss cheese	393	26,96	30,99	1,44	0	1,44	0
Yoghurt (Bulgarian, Greek, plain)	97	9	5	3,98	0	3,98	4
NUTS, UNBLANCHED, RAW							
Pecans	691	9,17	71,97	13,86	9,6	4,26	3,97
Brazil nuts, dried	659	14,32	67,1	11,74	7,55	4,19	2,33
SEEDS, WHOLE							
Flaxseeds/linseeds	534	18,29	42,16	28,88	27,3	1,58	1,55
Pumpkin seeds	559	30,23	49,05	10,71	6	4,71	1,4
All nuts and seeds should be activated.							
BEVERAGES							
Coffee (espresso); leaf teas	9	0,12	0,18	1,67	0	1,67	0
Coconut water unsweetened (from green coconuts)	19	0,72	0,2	3,71	1,1	2,61	2,61
Beers, cider	43	0	0	3,55	0	3,55	0
Alcohol (gin, rum, vodka, whisky)	250	0	0	0,1	0	0,1	0
Wine, red	85	0,07	0	2,61	0	2,61	0,62
Wine, Rosé	83	0,36	0	3,8	0	3,8	3,8
Wine, white, Sauvignon Blanc	82	0,07	0	2,27	0	2,27	2,27
Wine, white, Pinot Gris	83	0,07	0	2,06	0	2,06	2,06
Wine, white, Chenin Blanc	80	0,07	0	3,31	0	3,31	-
Note on alcohol: this will slow weight loss and is a toxin; regular use is not encouraged.							

All animal meats, beef, lamb, chicken, pork and game are allowed. Must be free from marinades, and preferably hormone-free and humanely treated.

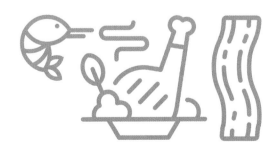

THE ORANGE LIST

FRUIT	CALORIES	PROTEIN	TOTAL FAT	CARBS	FIBRE	NET CARBS	SUGAR
Apples	52	0,26	0,17	13,81	2,4	11,41	10,39
Apricots	48	1,4	0,39	11,12	2	9,12	9,1
Bananas	89	1,09	0,33	22,84	2,6	20,24	12,23
Blueberries	57	0,74	0,33	14,49	2,4	12,09	9,96
Cherries, sour	50	1	0,3	12,18	1,6	10,58	8,49
Cherries, sweet	63	1,06	0,2	16,01	2,1	13,91	12,82
Clementines	47	0,85	0,15	12,02	1,7	10,32	9,18
Cranberries, fresh	46	0,46	0,13	11,97	3,6	8,37	4,27
Currants, red and white	56	1,4	0,2	13,8	4,3	9,5	7,37
Elderberries	73	0,66	0,5	18,4	7	11,4	11,4
Figs	74	0,75	0,3	19,18	2,9	16,28	16,26
Gooseberries	44	0,88	0,58	10,18	4,3	5,88	-
Grapefruit	32	0,63	0,1	8,08	1,1	6,98	6,98
Grapes	69	0,72	0,16	18,1	0,9	17,2	15,48
Guavas	68	2,55	0,95	14,32	5,4	8,92	8,92
Kiwifruit	61	1,14	0,52	14,66	3	11,66	8,99
Kumquats	71	1,88	0,86	15,9	6,5	9,4	9,36
Lemons without peel	29	1,1	0,3	9,32	2,8	6,52	2,5
Limes	30	0,7	0,2	10,54	2,8	7,74	1,69
Loquats	47	0,43	0,2	12,14	1,7	10,44	-
Lychees	66	0,83	0,44	16,53	1,3	15,23	15,23
Mangos	60	0,82	0,38	14,98	1,6	13,38	13,66
Melons	36	0,54	0,14	9,09	0,8	8,29	8,12
Mulberries	43	1,44	0,39	9,8	1,7	8,1	8,1
Nectarines	44	1,06	0,32	10,55	1,7	8,85	7,89

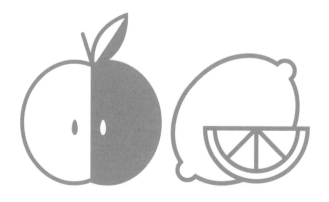

THE ORANGE LIST

FRUIT	CALORIES	PROTEIN	TOTAL FAT	CARBS	FIBRE	NET CARBS	SUGAR
Oranges	47	0,94	0,12	11,75	2,4	9,35	9,35
Passion fruit/granadilla	97	2,2	0,7	23,38	10,4	12,98	11,2
Pawpaw/papaya	43	0,47	0,26	10,82	1,7	9,12	7,82
Peaches	39	0,91	0,25	9,54	1,5	8,04	8,39
Pears	57	0,36	0,14	15,23	3,1	12,13	9,75
Pineapples	50	0,54	0,12	13,12	1,4	11,72	9,85
Plums	46	0,7	0,28	11,42	1,4	10,02	9,92
Pomegranates	83	1,67	1,17	18,07	4	14,07	13,67
Prickly pears	41	0,73	0,51	9,57	3,6	5,97	-
Quinces	57	0,4	0,1	15,3	1,9	13,4	-
Raspberries	52	1,2	0,65	11,94	6,5	5,44	4,42
Strawberries	32	0,67	0,3	7,68	2	5,68	4,89
Tangerines	53	0,81	0,31	13,34	1,8	11,54	10,58
Watermelon	30	0,61	0,15	7,55	0,4	7,15	6,2
NUTS, UNBLANCHED, RAW							
Almonds	579	21,15	49,93	21,55	12,5	9,05	4,35
Almond butter	614	20,96	55,5	18,82	10,3	8,52	4,43
Coconut desiccated, unsweetened	660	6,88	64,53	23,65	16,3	7,35	7,35
Coconut flesh	354	3,33	33,49	15,23	9	6,23	6,23
Hazelnuts	628	14,95	60,75	16,7	9,7	7	4,34
Macadamia nuts	718	7,91	75,77	13,82	8,3	5,52	4,57
Pine nuts	673	13,69	68,37	13,08	3,7	9,38	3,59
Pistachios	560	20,16	45,32	27,17	10,6	16,57	7,66
Tahini, sesame butter	586	18,08	50,87	24,05	5,5	18,55	-
Walnuts, English	654	15,23	65,21	13,71	6,7	7,01	2,61

All nuts and seeds should be preferably activated from raw nuts and seeds for superior absorption.

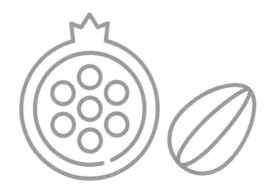

THE ORANGE LIST

SEEDS	CALORIES	PROTEIN	TOTAL FAT	CARBS	FIBRE	NET CARBS	SUGAR
Chia seeds	486	16,54	30,74	42,12	34,4	7,72	-
Caraway seeds	333	19,77	14,59	49,9	38	11,9	0,64
Poppy seeds	525	17,99	41,56	28,13	19,5	8,63	2,99
Sesame seeds	573	17,73	49,67	23,45	11,8	11,65	0,3
Sunflower seeds	584	20,78	51,46	20	8,6	11,4	2,62
VEGETABLES							
Arrowroot	65	4,24	0,2	13,39	1,3	12,09	-
Artichoke	47	3,27	0,15	10,51	5,4	5,11	0,99
Beets	43	1,61	0,17	9,56	2,8	6,76	6,76
Brussels sprouts	43	3,38	0,3	8,95	3,8	5,15	2,2
Butternut	45	1	0,1	11,69	2	9,69	2,2
Cabbage, red	31	1,43	0,16	7,37	2,1	5,27	3,83
Carrots	41	0,93	0,24	9,58	2,8	6,78	4,74
Celery root/celeriac	42	1,5	0,3	9,2	1,8	7,4	1,6
Dandelion leaves	45	2,7	0,7	9,2	3,5	5,7	0,71
Hearts of palm	115	2,7	0,2	25,61	1,5	24,11	17,6
Kale	49	4,28	0,93	8,75	3,6	5,15	2,26
Leeks	61	1,5	0,3	14,15	1,8	12,35	3,9
Onions	40	1,1	0,1	9,34	1,7	7,64	4,24
Parsnips	75	1,2	0,3	17,99	4,9	13,09	4,8
Peas, fresh, shelled, raw without pods (NB: this is technically a legume)	81	5,42	0,4	14,45	5,7	8,75	5,67
Peppermint herb, fresh	70	3,75	0,94	14,89	8	6,89	-
Peppers, yellow	27	1	0,21	6,32	0,9	5,42	-
Potatoes (not permitted on LCHF programmes)	77	2,05	0,09	17,49	2,1	15,39	0,82
Pumpkin	26	1	0,1	6,5	0,5	6	2,76
Seaweed, agar	26	0,54	0,03	6,75	0,5	6,25	0,28
Seaweed, kelp	43	1,68	0,56	9,57	1,3	8,27	0,6
Shallots	72	2,5	0,1	16,8	3,2	13,6	7,87
Snow peas	42	3	0	14	5	9	6
Sweet potato	86	1,57	0,05	20,12	3	17,12	4,18
Tomato purée	38	1,65	0,21	8,98	1,9	7,08	4,83

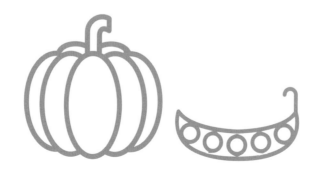

THE ORANGE LIST

DAIRY	CALORIES	PROTEIN	TOTAL FAT	CARBS	FIBRE	NET CARBS	SUGAR
Cream cheese, full fat	350	6,15	34,44	5,52	0	5,52	3,76
Milk, buffalo	97	3,75	6,89	5,18	0	5,18	5,18
Milk, sheep	108	5,98	7	5,36	0	5,36	-
CONDIMENTS, HERBS AND SPICES							
Balsamic vinegar	88	0,49	0	17,03	0	17,03	14,95
Basil, dried	233	22,98	4,07	47,75	37,7	10,05	1,71
Chilli powder	282	13,46	14,28	49,7	34,8	14,9	7,19
Chillies, hot pepper, red	40	1,87	0,44	8,81	1,5	7,31	5,3
Cocoa powder, unsweetened	228	19,6	13,7	57,9	37	20,9	1,75
Fennel seed	345	15,8	14,87	52,29	39,8	12,49	-
Ginger root	80	1,82	0,75	17,77	2	15,77	1,7
Horseradish, prepared	48	1,18	0,69	11,29	3,3	7,99	7,99
Lemon juice to flavour	22	0,35	0,24	6,9	0,3	6,6	2,52
Lemon peel, rind	47	1,5	0,3	16	10,6	5,4	4,17
Lime juice	25	0,42	0,07	8,42	0,4	8,02	1,69
Mustard powder	508	26,08	36,24	28,09	12,2	15,89	6,79
Paprika	282	14,14	12,89	53,99	34,9	19,09	10,34
Parsley, dried	292	26,63	5,48	50,64	26,7	23,94	7,27
Rosemary, fresh	131	3,31	5,86	20,7	14,1	6,6	-
Rosemary dried	331	4,88	15,22	64,06	42,6	21,46	-
Sage, dried	315	10,63	12,75	60,73	40,3	20,43	1,71
Thyme, fresh	101	5,56	1,68	24,45	14	10,45	-
Tomato paste	82	4,32	0,47	18,91	4,1	14,81	12,18
Vanilla extract	288	0,06	0,06	12,65	0	12,65	12,65
Wasabi root, raw	109	4,8	0,63	23,54	7,8	15,74	-
Worcestershire sauce	78	0	0	19,46	0	19,46	19,46

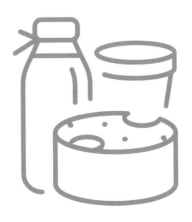

THE RED LIST

NUTS, UNBLANCHED, RAW	CALORIES	PROTEIN	TOTAL FAT	CARBS	FIBRE	NET CARBS	SUGAR
European chestnuts	196	1,63	1,25	44,17	5	39,17	-
Cashew nuts	553	18,22	43,85	30,19	3,3	26,89	5,91
STARCHY VEGETABLES, FRUIT AND DRIED FRUIT							
Apples, dried	243	0,93	0,32	65,89	8,7	57,19	57,19
Bananas, dried	519	2,3	33,6	58,4	7,7	50,7	35,34
Blueberries, dried	317	2,5	2,5	80	7,5	72,5	67,5
Chillies, dried	324	10,58	5,81	69,86	28,7	41,16	41,06
Dates, Medjool	277	1,81	0,15	74,97	6,7	68,27	66,47
Figs, dried	249	3,3	0,93	63,87	9,8	54,07	47,92
Garlic, fresh	149	6,36	0,5	33,06	2,1	30,96	1
Goji berries, dried	349	14,26	0,39	77,06	13	64,06	45,61
Mango, dried	319	2,45	1,18	78,58	2,4	76,18	66,27
Mushrooms, shiitake, dried	296	9,58	0,99	75,37	11,5	63,87	2,21
Peaches, dried	239	3,61	0,76	61,33	8,2	53,13	41,74
Pears, dried	262	1,87	0,63	69,7	7,5	62,2	62,2
Plums, dried	240	2,18	0,38	63,88	7,1	56,78	38,13
Raisins, seedless	299	3,07	0,46	79,18	3,7	75,48	59,19
Seaweed, dried	306	6,21	0,3	80,88	7,7	73,18	2,97
Tomato, sundried	258	14,11	2,97	55,76	12,3	43,46	37,59
SWEETENERS							
Chocolate, dark (commercial 70-85%)	625	7,5	47,5	42,5	7,5	35	30
Coconut sugar	375	0	0	100	0	100	95
Honey, raw, never commercial	304	0,3	0	82,4	0,2	82,2	82,12
Malt syrups	318	6,2	0	71,3	0	71,3	71,3
Maple syrup, Canadian	270	0	0	67,38	0	67,38	59,92
Molasses	290	0	0,1	74,73	0	74,73	74,72
DAIRY SUBSTITUTES							
Coconut cream, sweetened	357	1,17	16,13	53,21	0,2	53,01	51,5
CONDIMENTS, SPICES AND HERBS (IN LIMITED QUANTITIES ALL MAY BE USED TO FLAVOUR FOODS)							
Spices (pure – no cornflour fillers in powders)							
Allspice, ground	263	6,09	8,69	72,12	21,6	50,52	-
Aniseed	337	17,6	15,9	50,02	14,6	35,42	-
Bay leaf	313	7,61	8,36	74,97	26,3	48,67	-
Cardamom, ground	311	10,76	6,7	68,47	28	40,47	-
Cayenne pepper	318	12,01	17,27	56,63	27,2	29,43	10,34
Cinnamon, ground	247	3,99	1,24	80,59	53,1	27,49	2,17
Cloves, ground	274	5,97	13	65,53	33,9	31,63	2,38
Coriander leaf, dried	279	21,93	4,78	52,1	10,4	41,16	41,16
Cumin seed	375	17,81	22,27	44,24	10,5	33,74	2,25
Garlic powder	331	16,55	0,73	72,73	9	63,73	2,43
Ginger, ground	335	8,98	4,24	71,62	14,1	57,52	3,39

THE RED LIST

	CALORIES	PROTEIN	TOTAL FAT	CARBS	FIBRE	NET CARBS	SUGAR
CONDIMENTS, SPICES AND HERBS (IN LIMITED QUANTITIES ALL MAY BE USED TO FLAVOUR FOODS)							
Mace, ground	475	6,71	32,38	50,5	20,2	30,3	-
Nutmeg, ground	525	5,84	36,31	49,29	20,8	28,49	2,99
Onion powder	341	10,41	1,04	79,12	15,2	63,92	6,63
Oregano, dried	265	9	4,28	68,92	42,5	26,42	4,09
Pepper, black	251	10,39	3,26	63,95	25,3	38,65	0,64
Pepper, white	296	10,4	2,12	68,61	26,2	42,41	0
Saffron	310	11,43	5,85	65,37	3,9	61,47	-
Tarragon, dried	295	22,77	7,24	50,22	7,4	42,82	-
Thyme, dried	276	9,11	7,43	63,94	37	26,94	1,71
Turmeric, dried powder	312	9,68	3,25	67,14	22,7	44,44	3,21
Wasabi root	292	2,23	10,9	46,13	6,1	40,3	13,2

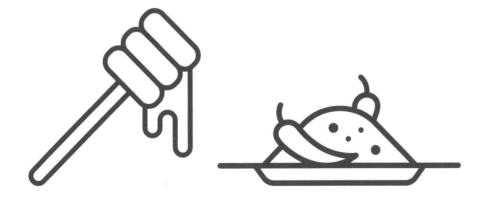

THE BANNED LIST

MEATS
Basted meats (often contains sugar and MSG)
Polony
Processed meats
Salami (unless made the old-fashioned healthy way)
Tinned meats in sugars
All soya meats or meats containing grain

FATS AND OILS
Blended oils (canola and olive oil blends) and hydrogenated oils
Canola oil
Flaxseed oil
Grapeseed oil
Hemp oil
Soyabean oil
Margarine
Pomace oil
Safflower oil
Sunflower oil
Vegetable fats and oils

DAIRY
Dairy powders
Flavoured drinking yoghurts
Flavoured milkshakes
Processed cheeses (wrapped cheese wedges, sandwich cheeses)
Ice cream, frozen yoghurts
All low-fat, lite, reduced fat, fat-free products

PROCESSED, CANNED AND BAKED FOODS
Processed salad dressings and bastings
Processed sauces
Tinned pastas
Tinned vegetables and soups

CONFECTIONERY AND BAKED GOODS
Biscuits
Bread of any kind
Cereals of any kind
Cornflour and wheat flours
Cakes with refined flours
Corn and rice cakes
Gluten-free refined baked goods
Muffins, flapjacks, biscotti, etc

SWEETENERS AND FLAVOURANTS
Acesulfame K, Cyclamates
Agave
Aspartame
Benzoic acid
Brominated vegetable oil
Cycalmates and saccharin
Dextrose
Fructose
High fructose corn syrup
Isomalt
MSG
Nature identical flavourings – these are not natural, they are chemicals
Potassium metabisulphite
Potassium sorbate
Sucralose
Sugars (brown, white)
Unnatural (chemical) preservatives

BEVERAGES
Commercial flavoured waters
Commercial cordials
Energy drinks
Fruit juices (commercial)
Instant coffees and shakes; tinned powdered drinks
Restaurant powdered smoothies and coffees (must be naturally made)
Sodas, fizzy drinks, soft drinks

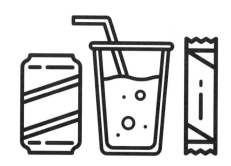

THE BANNED LIST

GRAINS, LEGUMES AND BEANS	NET CARBS
Amaranth	58.55
Barley, pearled	62.12
Buckwheat	61.5
Bulgar	63.37
Chickpeas	50.75
Corn white, yellow, fresh, sweetcorn	66.96
Couscous	72.43
Lentils	52.65
Millet	64.35
Oat bran	50.82
Oats	55.67
Pasta (all grain-based pasta)	71.47
Peanuts	7.00
Polenta, non-GMO	69.59
Popcorn, air popped, non-GMO, not in a microwave	63.28
Quinoa	57.16
Rice flour	77.73
Rice, brown, medium grain	72.77
Rice, white, medium grain	77.94
Rye grain	60.76
Semolina	68.93
Sorghum	65.39
Soya	varies
Spelt	59.49
Split peas	38.24
Tamarind	57.4
Teff	65.13

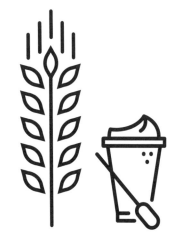

You will find foods that low-carb adherents do not and should not eat from this Banned list (hence the name). What we would like to draw your attention to is the grains, legumes and beans section of this list. While we don't recommend grains or legumes at all at any time for Paleo/low-carb lifestylers, we need to show these somewhere and short of creating another list, we have chosen to put them into this Banned list. We have included their carb amounts for the sake of other family members who may not be low-carb/Paleo, but who wish to know the strict carb counts of some of these foods.

06

LET'S EAT!

In cooking you've got to have a 'what the hell' attitude.

– Julia Child

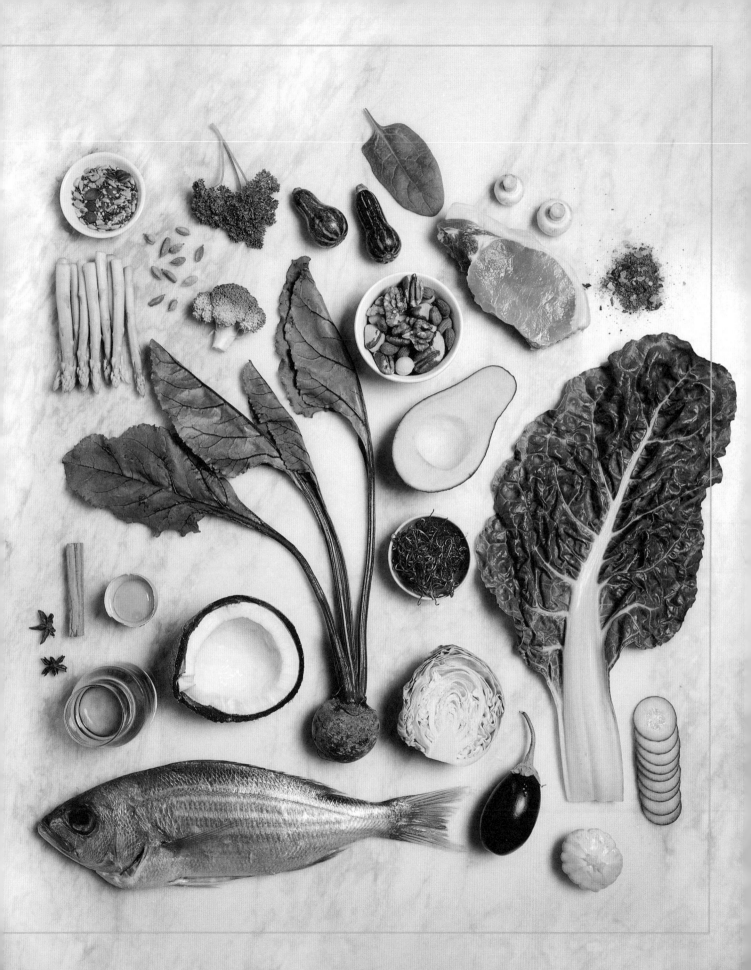

Chapter

06

BASIC COOKING TECHNIQUES

It's not surprising that there are so many people who lack basic cooking skills. In many families, both parents often work, and with so little time, they have no idea how long to roast a chicken or even how to boil an egg – essential skills that everyone should know. If you want to be healthy, you have to learn to cook. Not fine dining, but the fundamentals. Often, people can follow complex recipes and produce gourmet food for dinner parties, yet are lost when it comes to the basics. Converting to a low-carb lifestyle means getting back to basics, and you can enjoy making many things your mother and grandmother made. It used to be taken for granted that you would learn most of these skills at home, but this is no longer the case. So let's get back to basics, and teach our children how to cook in the process.

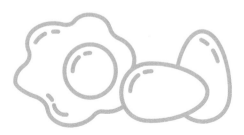

EGGS.

Boiled eggs

For perfectly soft-boiled eggs, bring a pan of water to the boil and then lower room-temperature eggs carefully into the water with a spoon so they don't break. Simmer for three and a half minutes for a medium-sized egg and four minutes for a large one. For hard-boiled eggs, place the eggs into cold water in the pan and bring to the boil. Reduce the heat and start timing once it begins to simmer: medium-sized eggs take nine minutes and larger eggs take 10 minutes. Plunge the eggs into cold water to stop the cooking process. This makes it easier to remove the shell, too.

Omelette

Break the amount of eggs you wish to use (depending on how many people you are feeding) into a bowl and add 30ml water for every four eggs used. Now mix the eggs and water with a fork or whisk, and season with salt and pepper. Heat your pan and melt 15g of butter in the pan. Pour the egg mixture into the pan and stir gently until it starts to set. Now pull the sides of the omelette away from the side of the pan gently so that the raw egg from the top can cook. As soon as it is set, you can add a filling on to half of the omelette, fold it in half, and serve.

Poached eggs

Fill a saucepan three-quarters full with water and simmer. Add 15ml of vinegar to the water. Break an egg into a cup, and slide it into the simmering water carefully. It takes three to four minutes to poach, after which you can remove it carefully with a slotted spoon.

Scrambled eggs

Break eggs into a bowl and mix them with a fork. Add 15ml of cream or water for every two eggs used. Season with salt and pepper. Melt some butter (20g for two eggs) in a frying pan over low heat. Pour in the egg mixture and stir gently until the consistency is thick and creamy.

CHICKEN.

Roast chicken is one of the easiest meals to make. Try to roast an extra chicken at the same time so that it can be used for lunch boxes, added to salads or shredded over zoodles or cabbage for another meal.

Roast chicken

Choose the best chicken you can afford, free range or organic is first prize. Heat your oven to 200°C. Brush the skin with melted butter, duck fat or lard. Grease the roasting tin with butter or lard, and put the chicken into it. Season the chicken with salt and pepper. If you want gravy, you can add a cup of chicken stock and a glass of white wine to the pan, this can be seasoned and used as sauce. Work on 20 minutes per 500g for cooking time.

Chicken livers

These are an easy option if you are looking to add extra protein to anything. Flash fry in a pan or grill. Please see page 180 for instructions.

Chicken pieces

Great to grill or barbecue, these only take 20 to 25 minutes to cook. Save all the bones from your chicken, even if you need to freeze them until you have enough; they can be used to make a stock.

Easy stock

Make stock from chicken bones, using the carcasses of three chickens or more. Place them in a big pot with a stick of celery, a couple of cut carrots, one onion quartered, a couple of bay leaves, some sprigs of parsley – including the stalks – and six peppercorns. Cover with cold water and add 15ml of apple cider vinegar. Bring to a boil and then turn down to simmer gently for about four hours. Once it's done, strain off the liquid and use this as your stock. Divide it into serving sizes and freeze for later use. It's quite useful to freeze some in ice cube trays. Once they are frozen, remove them from the trays and store in a Ziploc bag. This makes it very easy to grab a few to add to any dish that calls for stock.

LAMB.

Lamb stew

A comforting, warming option – see notes on how to make a stew.

Lamb chops

Another family favourite, these are easy to barbecue or grill. Season them with salt and pepper, and grill until cooked to your liking.

Lamb curry

Fragrant and delicious – see curry recipe on page 166.

Lamb shanks

Pop them in an ovenproof dish, add a chopped onion, a couple of chopped carrots, a bay leaf or two, six peppercorns and some fresh herbs from your garden and cover the meat with some homemade stock (plus a glass or two of red wine if you wish). Seal the top of the dish well with foil or a tight-fitting lid, and bake at 180°C for the first hour, then turn the temperature down to 160°C and cook for another two to three hours, until the meat is tender.

Roast lamb

Lamb is particularly delicious roasted on a rack with water in the pan underneath which helps to keep the meat moist and tender. You could place a foil 'tent' over the meat and roast it long and slow. Roast your lamb under the tent at 160°C for four to five hours depending on the size of the roast. The meat won't be very pink, but it will be delicious. For a quicker option, preheat your oven to 200°C and then work out your timing according to how you like it cooked. For every 450g of meat, cook for 18 minutes for rare, 24 minutes for medium and 28 to 30 minutes for well done.

BEEF.

Brisket and short rib

These fatty cuts are excellent. Fatty cuts of meat are full of flavour and inexpensive. Grill the brisket, or make a casserole. Short rib needs to be cooked for quite a bit longer, either in a 180°C oven on a rack seasoned with salt and pepper, or on the barbecue. Watch it and turn after about 15 minutes; the cooking time will vary according to your oven.

Without a sauce, steak isn't very flavoursome. However, brisket will become a firm favourite in your household if you cook it properly – it's a much cheaper cut of meat, and although a little tougher, it is very tasty.

Oxtail

Choose an ovenproof dish or roasting pan to pack in all your pieces tightly. The bone will be touching the bottom of your dish. Now add a sliced onion, a punnet of sliced mushrooms, some bay leaves and a few peppercorns. You could cover the meat with stock or red wine; all the alcohol will cook away and you will be left with the most amazing flavour. Now seal the top tightly with foil, and cook it for four to five hours at 160°C. Check on how it's doing from time to time – the little end caps on the bone will be coming off when it is done.

Roast beef

If you wish to roast beef, look for rib, sirloin or topside. You need a piece of meat with a decent amount of fat on it (no more lean, boring, meat for low-carbers). Calculate your cooking time per 500g like this: 15 minutes for every 500g for rare and 20 minutes per 500g for well done. This applies to meat on the bone. If it has been deboned, add an extra five minutes to your cooking time.

Pot roast

Pot roasts are so easy to make. Use rolled topside or top rib or brisket. First preheat your oven to 170°C. Now brown your meat in lard or tallow in an ovenproof casserole dish – use one that can be used on the stove top as well as in the oven.

Once it is browned, remove the meat and set aside. Now sauté together one finely chopped onion, one large carrot finely chopped, two finely chopped celery stalks and one clove of crushed garlic, until soft. Add 300ml of red wine or homemade stock, a tin of tomatoes, a bay leaf and some salt and pepper. Place the meat back into the casserole dish, close the lid and bake in the oven for about three hours. Turn once during cooking. Once cooked, set aside the joint. Remove the bay leaf and use a hand-held blender to turn all the bits and the pan juices into a really tasty sauce to serve with the meat.

Steak

To cook steak, you need a really hot pan, or grill (or use the grill on a gas barbecue, as the grills on most ovens don't reach the required temperature). If your pan isn't hot enough, you will be stewing the meat, so get your pan really hot. Now you can sear the meat; cook it on one side and then turn it to cook the other side. Don't prod it with a fork – you don't want to lose all those wonderful juices.

PORK.

Pork belly

Pork belly has to be one of the most delectable cuts of meat. Buy it rolled and cook it slowly for a long time. I always cook extra to set aside. Put the pork belly on an oven rack, with some water in a pan underneath. 'Tent' with foil and cook at 170°C for four to five hours. Once the meat is tender, take it out the oven and turn on the grill. Remove the foil and grind some salt over the skin.

Now place it under the grill to get the crackling wonderfully crispy. Watch it very carefully as you don't want to burn it. When you use the leftover belly roll, cut into slices and sauté it in a pan. The fat will crisp up and you will have delicious slices of meat to serve with vegetables or salad.

Pork chops and steaks

These can be fried or grilled. If you fry them, add a spoonful of any kind of dripping to your hot pan, sear both sides of the meat to seal in the juices. Turn the pan down and cook at a lower temperature until cooked through. To grill, put your oven shelf close to the element, grill until the meat is brown and then turn over and do the same on the other side. If your piece of meat is fairly thin, it will probably cook quite quickly, otherwise turn the oven down and continue cooking a while longer until done.

Trotters

These also make a great meal – see the recipe on page 177.

SEAFOOD.

Baked fish

You can either bake fish in a dish, or in foil. If using a dish, grease the bottom of the dish, add the fish and season it with salt, black pepper, fresh lemon or lime juice and dot with butter. Cover the dish and bake. You could ask your fishmonger for cooking times according to the type of fish you

have purchased – even the fish counters in supermarkets will have someone who is able to help you with this.

If you are baking in foil, smear the foil with butter to stop the fish from sticking to it. If you have a whole fish, it's a good idea to put slices of lemon in the middle to infuse the flesh with a lovely lemony taste. Season it with salt and pepper and dot with butter. Wrap up the parcel tightly and bake in the oven or on the braai – it makes a wonderful meal done on a braai.

Grilled fish

This is also an easy option. Brush the fish with butter and season with salt and pepper. Watch carefully while the fish is under the grill to avoid overcooking.

Pan-fried fish

Pan-fried fish is traditionally coated in seasoned flour; you can use ground almonds or desiccated coconut instead. Fry in plenty of butter, and then season with salt and pepper and serve with lemon wedges.

Crayfish

This delicacy is delicious cooked on the barbecue, and even better when freshly caught. To prepare crayfish, you need a very sharp knife, or a really good pair of kitchen scissors. Start at the tail end, and cut up the centre of the back, cutting through the shell. Go straight up the back from the tail into the head, up between the eyes, between the feelers, down between the mouth and the middle of the area between the legs. Continue down, cutting through the thin membrane-like covering on the underside of the tail, until you get to your starting point at the end of the tail.

Now use a knife to cut the crayfish in half. Remove the intestine that runs down the length of the tail, and the mustard-coloured innards in the head area. Barbecue meat-side down for five minutes then turn over and baste liberally with a homemade butter, lemon, garlic and chilli mixture. Cook until the flesh is white throughout. The total cooking time should be no more than 15 minutes.

Calamari

Calamari steaks are perfect; just fry in some butter and serve with lemon and garlic. Tubes can be fried, or even added to a tomato-based sauce. Both are equally delicious and very easy to cook.

Prawns

Try to source prawns that have already been deveined. Then simply butterfly the prawns, brush the flesh with a mixture of butter, lemon juice and crushed garlic, and grill. As soon as the flesh turns white, your prawns are cooked.

VEGETABLES.

Gem squash

These can be cut in half and steamed. Then remove the pips and serve with butter. Or fill them with cooked mince, top with cheese and grill them in the oven or bake them for 15 minutes.

Steaming

This is a very healthy way to cook vegetables until they are just tender and they will not lose any flavour. Do yourself a favour and buy a stainless steel steamer that can fit into several of your pots. Add water underneath the steamer and bring it to the boil, then turn it down to simmer. Cut the vegetables to the size you want them and steam until tender. See our recipes for some ideas on how to jazz up your vegetables once they are steamed.

Stir-frying

This method is a quick way to cook vegetables. Use a wok or a large frying pan. Put coconut oil or animal fat in the pan, get it smoking hot and the fry your veggies till just cooked.

Roast vegetables

This is always a winner, and so easy to prepare. You can cook extra roast vegetables as they are delicious when cold, and can be added to salads, or warmed up for a quick meal. Even pop some in your child's lunchbox. Use any combination of onion, coloured peppers, aubergines, whole button mushrooms, courgettes, green beans, whole cloves of garlic in their skin (delicious squeezed out once cooked), pattypans, baby gems squash or any other vegetables that you may wish to add. (If you are following a more Paleo approach, you could add in some carrot and sweet potato chunks.) Cut these into large chunks all about the same size, toss in some olive oil, melted duck fat or coconut oil, season with salt and pepper and roast at 180°C till the vegetables are done. Some of them will caramelise at the corners, which is even more delicious. This is an excellent side to any meat, fish or chicken dish.

HOW TO MAKE A STEW.

Stews can be prepared with any type of meat, poultry or fish. The joy of making a stew is that once you have done the preparation, you can leave it to cook and go off and do something else. The longer the stew cooks, the more tender the meat will be, and stewing meats are usually the cheapest cuts of meat – you win both ways. You can also add a variety of vegetables to the pot and cook it gently and over a period of time in some homemade bone broth. For added flavour, you can add a splash of wine, but this is not necessary.

In order to make a really good stew, preparation is necessary. First brown the meat in a pot for the best flavour. Do this in batches; use lard and a high temperature to seal in those juices. You want the meat to be nicely browned, not a pale, insipid colour.

As you brown each batch of meat, remove it from your pot and season generously with Himalayan salt and ground black pepper. You may need to add more fat to the meat; this is fine. Building up a crust on the bottom of the pot will give your stew an amazing flavour.

Once all the meat is browned, add some extra lard to the pan and sauté a couple of chopped onions and a few chopped stalks of celery. Once the onion is translucent, add two cloves of crushed garlic, 30ml of tomato paste and stir well. Now is the time to deglaze your pot; place a cup of wine (usually red for red meat and white for chicken or fish) or a cup of broth into the pot and let it boil up nicely. As it starts to bubble, stir and scrape the sticky residue from the bottom of the pot (that's what deglazing means), it will dissolve into the liquid to give your stew a delicious flavour.

Add the meat back into the pot with a litre of broth as well as a bay leaf and some fresh herbs (thyme is particularly good). Reduce the heat to simmer, and cook for one and a half to two hours, stirring occasionally. Add some chopped carrots, sweet potatoes, mushrooms and any other vegetables you like, and cook for another hour. The meat should be tender. If not, just keep cooking. Taste your gravy, and add extra salt and pepper if needed. Once your preparation is done, you can also cook your stew in an oven casserole at 180°C, using times that are similar to the time for the stovetop. Alternatively, you can use a slow cooker.

Now you have absolutely no excuse. Recipes are only there to help you, so this should give you enough courage to get into the kitchen and rustle up a meal for the family.

Chapter

06
___

ALTERNATIVES TO FLOUR

People seem to miss bread terribly when they first go low-carb. But life can go on quite happily without your ever eating bread again. You learn to forget about bread. However, if you wanted some now and then, or need to bake, you could try one of the following flours.

COCONUT FLOUR.

Coconut flour is a very 'thirsty' flour, but it can make baking light and fluffy. It's naturally gluten-free, high in fibre and the healthiest alternative of all the flours. You could also use coconut flour to thicken stews and gravies. If you want to bake with it, use an equal amount of liquid to flour to prevent your dish drying out.

NUT AND SEED FLOURS.

A quarter cup of almond flour yields six grams of carbs and three grams fibre, so it's only three grams per quarter cup. Almond flour is versatile and gives a lovely taste to baking and food alike. You can use a variety of nut and seed flours; they all have similar results.

XANTHAN GUM.

This is a great natural replacement for gluten in baking, and is useful for holding things together. Xanthan is successful in gluten-free baking and low-carb baking.

Other alternatives to gluten include psyllium, flax and chia, but sometimes the taste and consistency interferes with the final product. While all these are replacements, none act in exactly the same way as gluten.

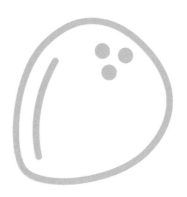

Chapter

06

ACTIVATING NUTS AND SEEDS

It's so much easier to buy ready-ground seed and nut flours today. For the most part, when you are stuck for time, it's fine. However, there's a dark side to nuts and seeds and their flours. Nuts and seeds should ideally be soaked, fully dehydrated and then eaten or made into flours. This may sound like something quite new and seemingly irrelevant, but it's rather important. Not only are they safer to eat, but they are so much tastier with more bioavailable nutrition.

If you have ever felt bloated after eating a muffin or piece of bread made from nut or seed flours, it's because the nuts or seeds were not activated first. By nature, nuts and seeds are very high in enzyme inhibitors, which cause bloating, gas and discomfort if they have not first been activated. Not everyone has the same degree of discomfort, but those who are sensitive battle with raw seeds and nuts. This is another reason why you should not consume these in large quantities on a daily basis; they should be eaten frugally.

Enzyme inhibitors like phytic acid and lectins are found in nuts and seeds. They bind important minerals in the body, including zinc, calcium, magnesium and manganese, preventing them from being available to the body. These enzyme inhibitors are there to prevent germination of the seed, which is no problem for the animals that eat them as they produce lots of the enzyme phytase to neutralise this phytic acid, but humans don't.

Soaking solves this by neutralising the phytic acid, and making the nutrients in the nuts and seeds more bioavailable to the body. This is something of a labour of love for your family, but the result is worth it.

Activating seeds and nuts means soaking them in warm water with salt for a period of time, rinsing and dehydrating them at a low temperature to preserve the delicate fats and nutrients.

The soaking times for nuts and seeds are all different; however, the following nuts and seeds will all require just seven hours of soaking. Rinse them well once soaked, and dry them at under 50 degrees Celsius to protect delicate oils.

- Almonds
- Hazelnuts
- Macadamia nuts
- Sunflower seeds
- Pecans
- Pine nuts
- Pumpkin seeds
- Walnuts

Dry them in a special dehydrator, and then store them in an airtight container. They will last well and taste amazing.

Roasted nuts are not the same as activated ones. Commercial nuts are generally deep fried in damaged fats and exposed to very high temperatures, which will denature their delicate fats, oxidising them. Make sure you dry the soaked nuts and seeds well to avoid mould growing on a damp surface. Activate your nuts and seeds and discover just how delicious they can be. But don't overeat them – they are tasty snacks and additions to meals, but shouldn't replace a meal.

AVOID TOO MANY SEED AND NUT FLOURS.

Low-carbers appear to be baking like crazy, and have tried every kind of treat known to man made with seed and nut flours, from breads to muffins, porridges, cakes, pizzas and everything in between. But did you know that you may be causing harm to yourself by having these flours daily? And maybe that's why you are no longer losing weight. There is a move to have more nuts and seeds, and their flours – but they are high in omega-6 fatty acids, which are inflammatory in excess, plus they are also full of anti-nutrients, unless activated first.

Concerns about excess nut and seed flours:

- A cup of almond flour equates to quite a lot of almonds – count them prior to grinding into flour. Eating them whole would limit your intake substantially, so try not to have too many.
- Almond flour is especially high in inflammatory polyunsaturated fatty acids (PUFA), around 20 per cent in fact. There are many reasons not to go overboard with PUFAs, as they:
  - Slow your metabolism
  - Are very inflammatory in larger amounts
  - Impair the action of certain digestive enzymes
  - Slow thyroid function
  - Inhibit detoxification enzymes
  - Deplete antioxidants in the body
  - Inhibit production of progesterone and androgens while activating production of oestrogen (a fat-building hormone which encourages oestrogen dominance) causing weight gain, PMS, hormonal acne and inflammation.
- While PUFAs aren't evil in small amounts, in large amounts they certainly are. This applies to all seed and nut flours – they should be pre-activated for good health.
- They're not that heat stable, and if not used, they may oxidise. That's why it's a good idea to buy nuts and seeds, activate them, and then grind them. Activating nuts and seeds properly will ensure you are not going to miss out on vital fats, minerals and other available nutrients.

Like everything in this low-carb lifestyle, excess should be avoided.

157

RECIPES

The only time to eat diet food is while you're waiting for the steak to cook.

– Julia Child

Please note: In the following recipes, 5ml = 1 tsp. We recommend that you have a good set of measuring spoons and cups indicating ml. Also note that a normal spoon in a cutlery set doesn't accurately measure 5ml.

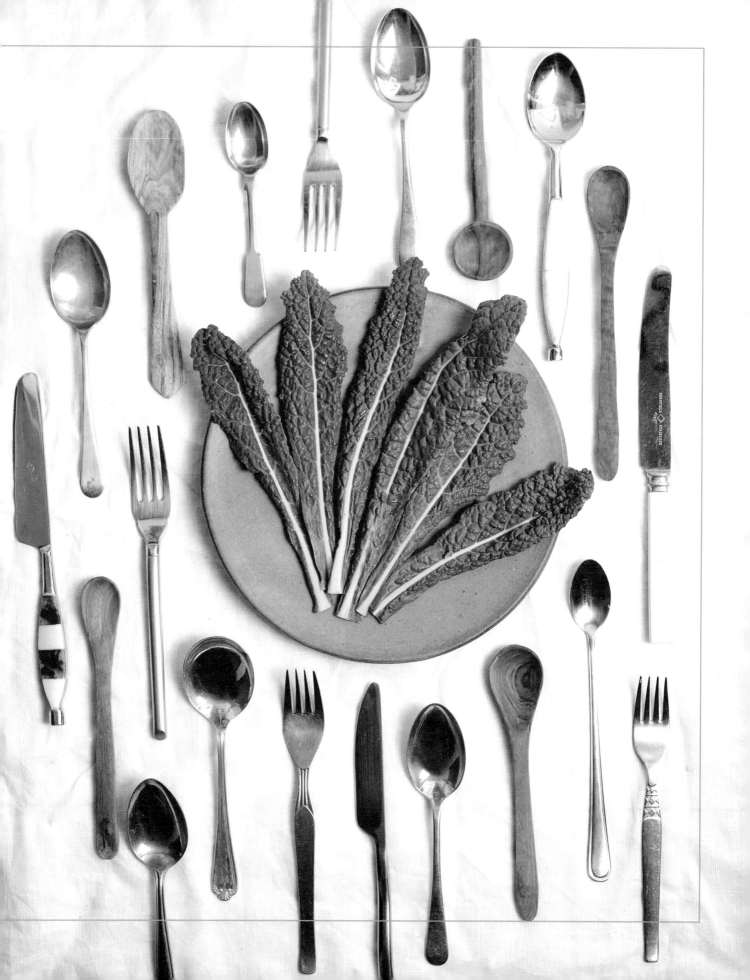

01

EGG MUFFINS

Serves 6

Egg muffins make a fantastic breakfast on the run. They can also be served with salad for lunch or popped into a lunch box. Delicious warm or cold.

INGREDIENTS

- 60g butter
- 1 onion, finely chopped
- 1 red pepper, finely chopped
- 250g mushrooms, sliced
- 1 clove of garlic, crushed
- 100g spinach, shredded
- 12 eggs
- Salt and pepper

METHOD

1. Preheat oven to 180°C. Grease a 12-hole muffin pan.
2. In a frying pan, melt the butter and sauté the onion and pepper until soft. Add the mushrooms and garlic and fry until the mushrooms are cooked through and all the fat has been absorbed. Stir the spinach into the mixture; it is not necessary to cook it.
3. Divide the vegetable mixture between the muffin cups.
4. Break all the eggs into a jug, whisk to combine, season with salt and pepper.
5. Divide the egg mixture evenly between the muffin cups. Give each one a stir to combine.
6. Bake for 15-20 minutes, until set.

VARIATIONS

- Add bacon or any other protein to the vegetable mixture.
- Vary the type of vegetables you use: courgettes, broccoli and cherry tomatoes are all good.
- Add some grated Cheddar or cubes of feta to the mixture.

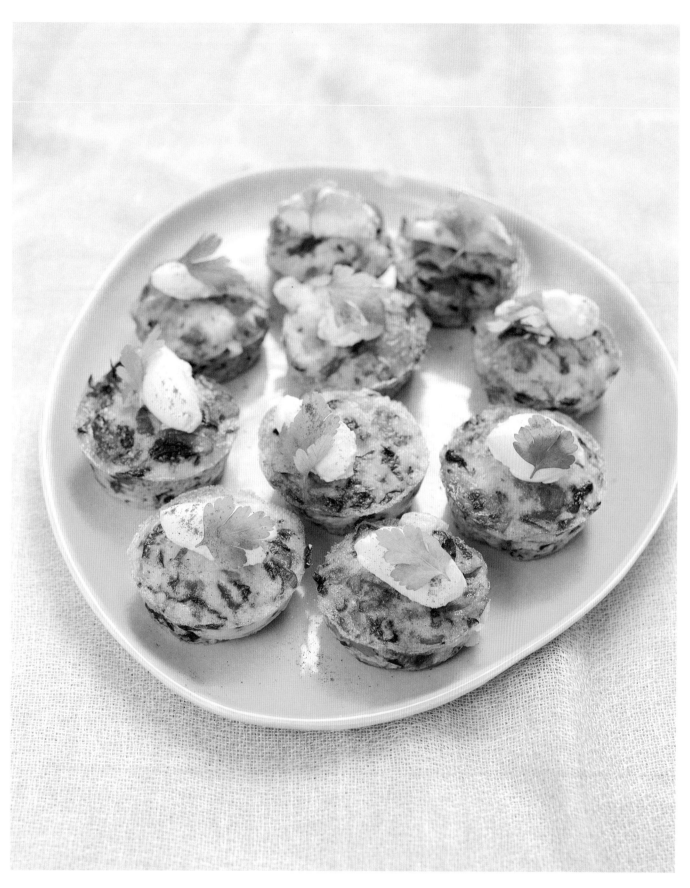

02

AUBERGINE STACK

Serves 2

This is a delightful and colourful way to have breakfast, or serve with salad for dinner or lunch.

INGREDIENTS

- 1 red pepper, deseeded and sliced into quarters
- 1 yellow pepper, deseeded and sliced into quarters
- 1 aubergine cut into 6 slices, about 5mm thick each
- 30ml olive oil
- 60ml Versatile Tomato Sauce (Recipe on p219)
- 1 tomato cut into 4-6 slices
- 8 basil leaves
- 4 slices of mozzarella cheese, 2-3mm thick
- Salt and pepper
- Poached egg to serve

METHOD

1. Preheat the oven to 180C.
2. Place the peppers onto a baking sheet and bake for 30 minutes.
3. Slice the aubergines into 5mm slices and sprinkle with salt. Set aside to sweat in a colander for about 15 minutes.
4. Rinse the aubergine thoroughly. Pat dry. Toss in a bowl with olive oil and some salt.
5. Heat a griddle pan on the stove till it is smoking hot.
6. Lay the aubergines on the griddle pan and grill for 2-3 minutes on each side until they become golden and slightly charred.
7. Set them aside on a paper towel and allow to drain.
8. Remove peppers from the oven. Allow the peppers to cool for a few minutes. You will have 4 red and 4 yellow slices.
9. Place 2 tbsp of tomato sauce onto a plate.
10. Lay a slice of aubergine in the middle of the tomato sauce, then top with a slice of tomato, 2 basil leaves, a slice of cheese and a slice of red, then yellow pepper. Repeat the pattern. Finish off with one more aubergine and a poached egg.

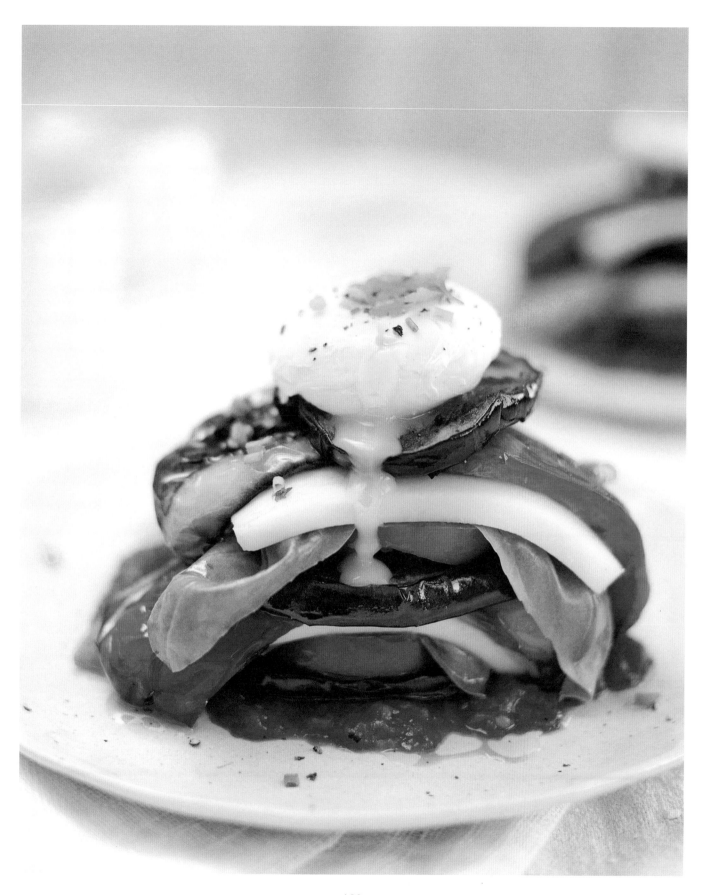

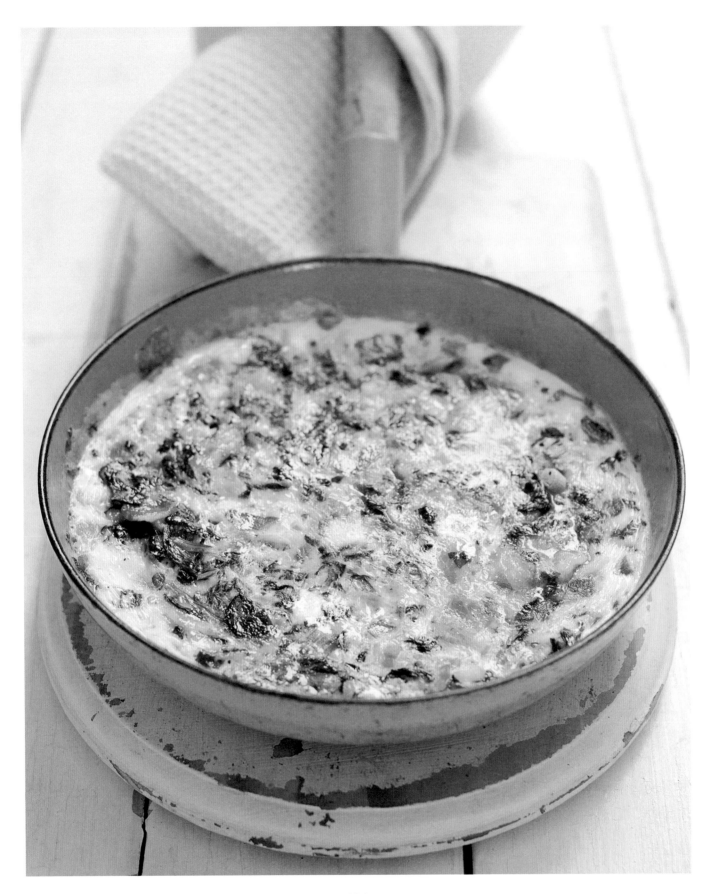

03

BACON AND SPINACH FRITTATA

Serves 4

Frittatas make a wonderful meal. They are perfect for breakfast, as leftovers they can be eaten cold, or you can even make one for a quick dinner. It's also a brilliant way to use up leftovers; be as creative as you like.

INGREDIENTS

- 30g of butter
- 100g of streaky bacon, chopped
- 200g spinach, shredded
- 4 spring onions, sliced
- 4 eggs
- Salt and pepper to taste

METHOD

1. Melt the butter in a pan, and then add the bacon and fry until cooked.
2. Add the spinach and allow it to wilt, along with the sliced spring onions.
3. Beat the eggs and season with salt and pepper, and pour the egg mixture into the pan.
4. Cook over a lower heat until the egg at the bottom of the pan has set.
5. You can put a lid on your pan and complete cooking on the stove, or put the pan under the grill to complete cooking.

VARIATIONS

- Chorizo with spinach or kale.
- Shredded cooked chicken and broccoli.
- Mince and any leftover vegetable.
- Cabbage with bacon (leftover cooked cabbage is perfect).
- Any combination of vegetables, fresh or leftover.
- Add cheese to the frittata: feta, Cheddar and blue cheese are all delicious.
- Tuna with any combination of vegetables you like.
- Mushroom and asparagus.

Mains **01**
___

CURRY

Serves 4

The secret to this recipe is that it uses real spices. The quantities can be increased but for every 500g of meat, add 100g of fat, and increase the spice accordingly. For cooking on a budget, use tripe. It is very nutritious and surprisingly delicious.

INGREDIENTS

- 100ml coconut oil
- 1 large onion, chopped
- ½ tsp turmeric
- 1 bay leaf
- 3 small cinnamon sticks
- 1 tbsp fennel seeds
- 1 sprig curry leaves
- 60ml masala
- 2 tsp ginger and garlic paste
- 1 tomato
- 500g mutton pieces (or lamb, chicken or tripe)
- 2 tsp salt
- 2 or 3 sweet potatoes, cubed
- Coriander, chopped

METHOD

1. Heat oil, add onion, turmeric and spices and fry to soften onion.
2. Add masala, ginger and garlic, and fry for a few seconds.
3. Add tomato – grating it works really well.
4. When the tomato is almost cooked, add meat and sauté.
5. Turn down the heat and cover. Make sure the meat is covered with liquid. Add water if necessary and cook until the meat is soft – a couple of hours at least.
6. Add the sweet potato and cook until tender.
7. Serve either on cauliflower rice or sautéed cabbage, garnished with coriander.

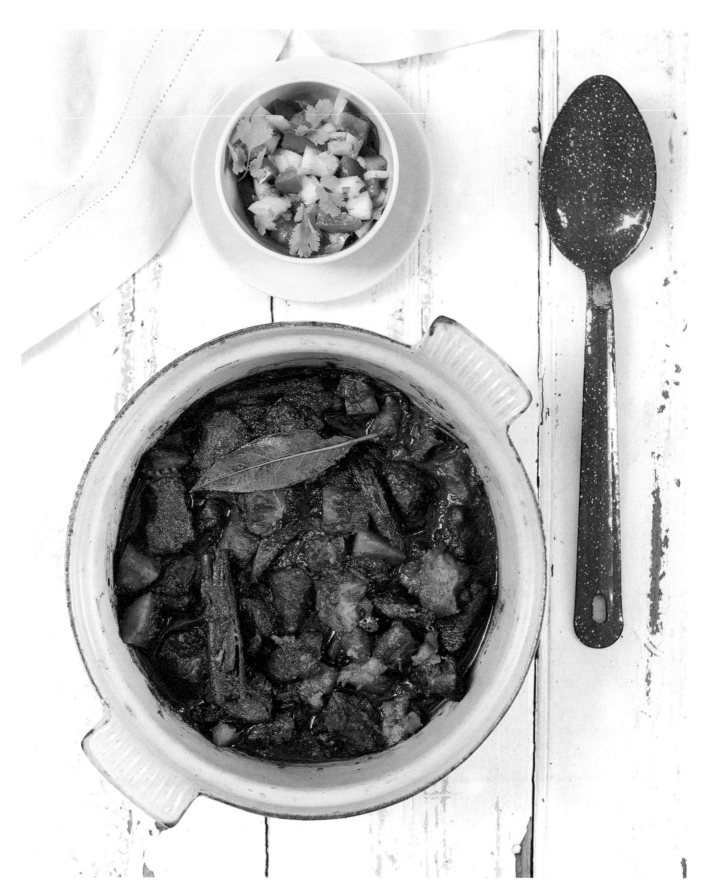

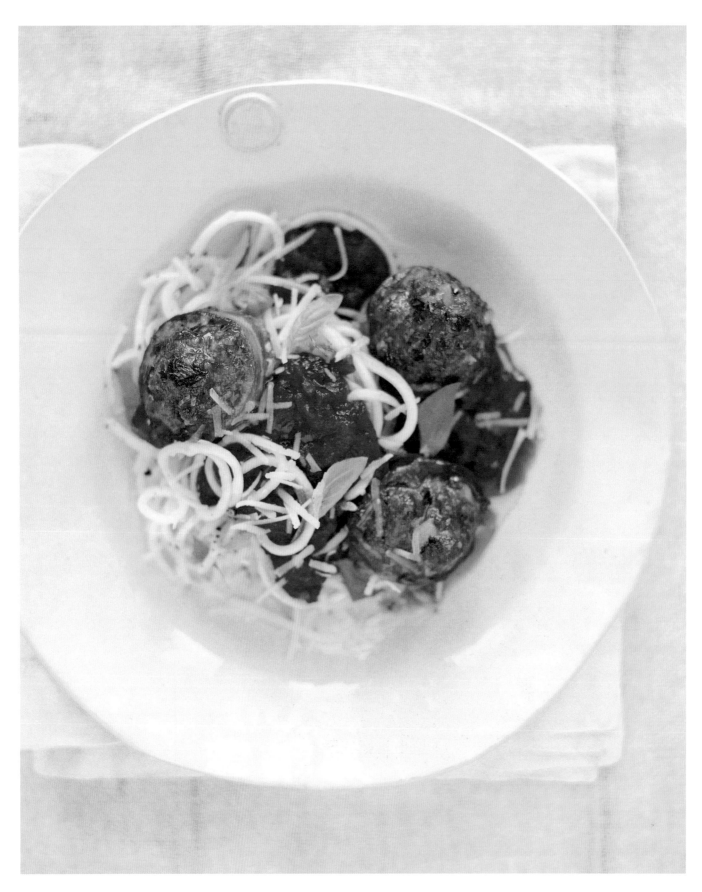

02

ZOODLES AND MEATBALLS Serves 4

A low-carb take on spaghetti and meatballs. The meatballs are also great alone or as a lunch box snack.

INGREDIENTS

- 480ml Versatile Tomato Sauce (see p219)
- 500g minced beef
- 200g bacon, cut into small chunks
- 8 additional strips of bacon
- 60ml coconut milk
- 2 cloves of garlic, minced
- 1 tsp mixed herbs
- ½ onion, grated
- Fresh parsley, chopped
- Ground black pepper
- 500g courgette zoodles
- 30g butter

METHOD

1. Prepare Versatile Tomato Sauce.
2. Preheat oven to 200°C.
3. In a big bowl, combine all the ingredients except the bacon strips, butter and the zoodles. Season with pepper.
4. Take a medium-sized muffin pan and place a slice of bacon around the sides of each hole.
5. Fill the holes with the beef mixture.
6. Cook for 30 minutes.
7. Toss the courgette zoodles in melted butter in a pan and fry until tender, but still firm.

TIP

Use smaller muffin pans to make double the quantity. You will need to slice the bacon strips in half, and adjust the cooking time.

Mains **03**

FISH PIE

Serves 6

This pie can be eaten hot or cold. This is a true budget meal that can feed half a dozen people if served with vegetables on the side. For a delicious twist, add cabbage fried in lard.

INGREDIENTS

- 400g tin of pilchards in brine
- 1 onion, chopped
- 2 tbsp coconut oil
- 2 tbsp coconut flour
- 3 eggs
- 250ml full cream milk
- 1 tsp salt
- Ground black pepper
- 1 tsp oregano

METHOD

1. Preheat oven to 180°C and grease a pie dish.
2. Drain the pilchards and mash them with a fork.
3. Lightly fry the onions in the coconut oil. Add the onion to the fish and stir.
4. Now add the coconut flour and eggs and stir well.
5. Lastly, add the milk and seasoning.
6. Pour all this into your pie dish and bake for 30 minutes.
7. The pie firms up on standing, so leave it for 10 minutes before slicing.

TIP

Add 250ml of grated Cheddar to the mixture. Add green pepper to the onion. You could also add chopped fresh parsley.

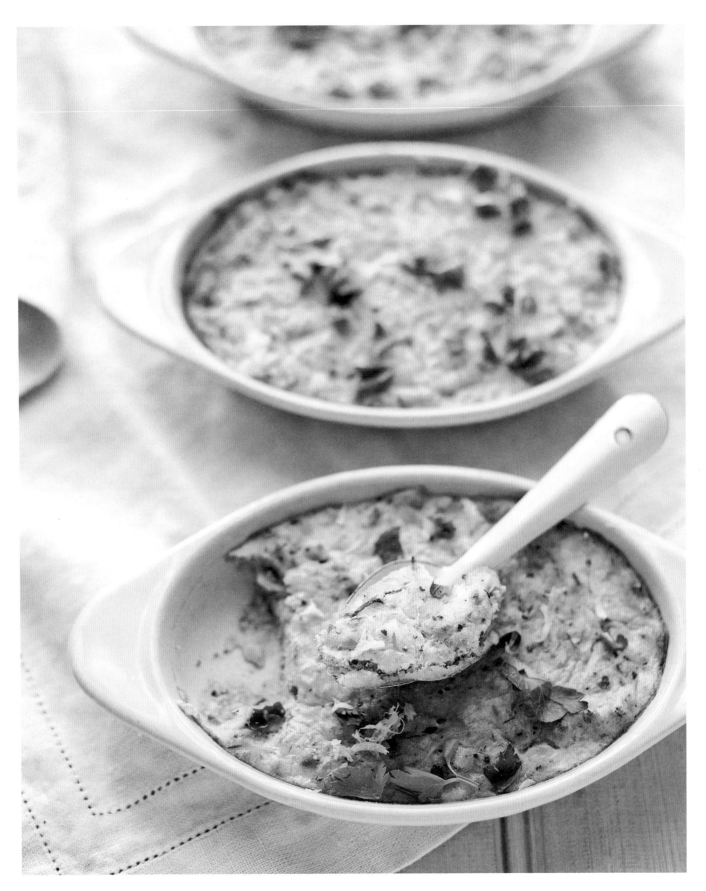

04

BRAWN

Makes 20-30 portions

Traditionally, brawn is made with a pig's head and as a result, is also called head cheese. I don't want to gross you out completely, so pork trotters have been substituted and work just as well. Brawn is a cold cut – basically a meat jelly – that originated in Europe. This version is made with ox tripe and pork trotters. The trotters provide the natural gelatine which allows the dish to set. It is best eaten cold or at room temperature, either with a salad or with some seed crackers or low-carb bread. This dish is packed with nutrition.

INGREDIENTS

- 4 pork trotters, cut into chunks
- 60ml coconut oil
- 2 onions, finely chopped
- 4-6 tbsp curry powder, adjust to taste
- 1½kg ox tripe, sliced thinly
- 1 litre of bone broth
- 125ml of vinegar
- 2 bay leaves
- Salt and pepper

METHOD

1. Place the trotters and tripe into a large ovenproof dish.
2. Melt the coconut oil and fry the onions until they are just translucent. Add the curry powder to the pan and fry for 1 minute; enjoy the wonderful curry aroma that emanates from the pan. Add this mixture to the dish with the trotters and tripe.
3. Warm the broth, add the vinegar and pour this over the mixture. The meat needs to be covered with liquid; if needed, top it up with water. Tuck the bay leaves into your dish.
4. Seal the dish tightly with aluminium foil or a lid, and cook at 180°C for an hour. Then turn down the oven to 120°C and cook for another 7 hours.
5. Be patient, as the mixture needs to be cool enough.
6. Now comes the messy bit. Scoop out the meat and remove all the bones with your hands. Chop all the meat from the trotters and the tripe into small pieces, and put them into a clean dish 37cm x 25cm; you can use more than one dish.
7. Season the meat with salt and pepper. Taste to make sure you have enough seasoning.
8. Strain the liquid through a sieve; you can use a spoon to push it through. Pour the liquid over the meat until it is completely covered.
9. Put this into the fridge to set. It sets very quickly as the liquid is full of gelatine.
10. Once set, cut it into portions and put some into the freezer for later use; it freezes particularly well.

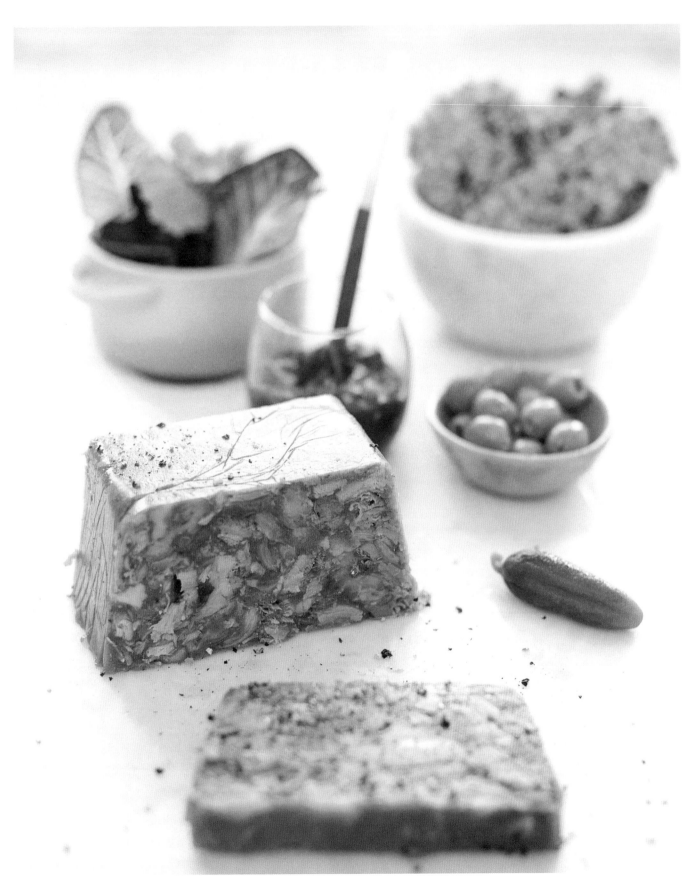

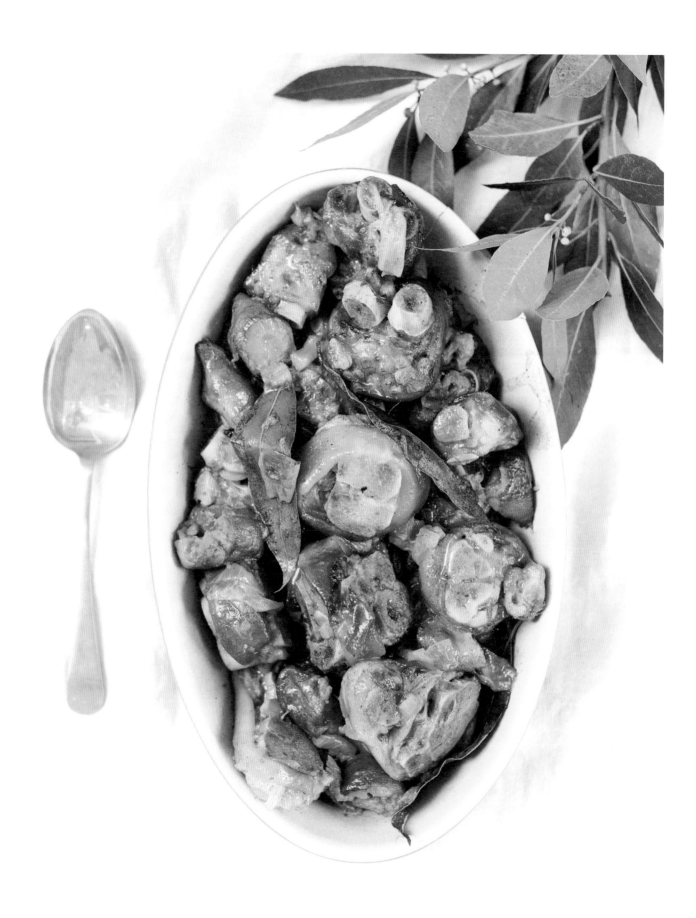

05

PORK TROTTERS

Serves 8-10

It is an excellent idea to cook extra trotters, as these are a wonderful source of gelatine and a truly affordable item. Any extra meat can be taken off the bone, chopped up and will set in the liquid to make brawn.

INGREDIENTS

- 4 pork trotters (ask the butcher to chop these into pieces for convenience, but don't panic if they are whole)
- 1 litre of bone broth
- The following ingredients are optional (for a real affordable recipe you can leave them all out except for the seasoning):
  - 2 bay leaves
  - 1 onion, chopped into quarters
  - 2 carrots, chopped into quarters
  - 8 peppercorns, or ground black pepper
  - Salt – add only at the end

METHOD

1. Put the trotters and all other ingredients into a roasting pan and cover with the broth. If the broth does not cover the trotters, top it up with water.
2. Use aluminium foil to seal the pan.
3. Cook at a moderate 150°C for 4-5 hours. The meat should be almost falling off the bone.
4. If you don't have an oven, it can be cooked on the stove at a low simmer. Make sure that the liquid does not dry out; you will need to add extra water, and this will take 3-4 hours.
5. You can also make this in a slow cooker.
6. Serve on shredded cooked cabbage, cauli-rice or cauli-mash.

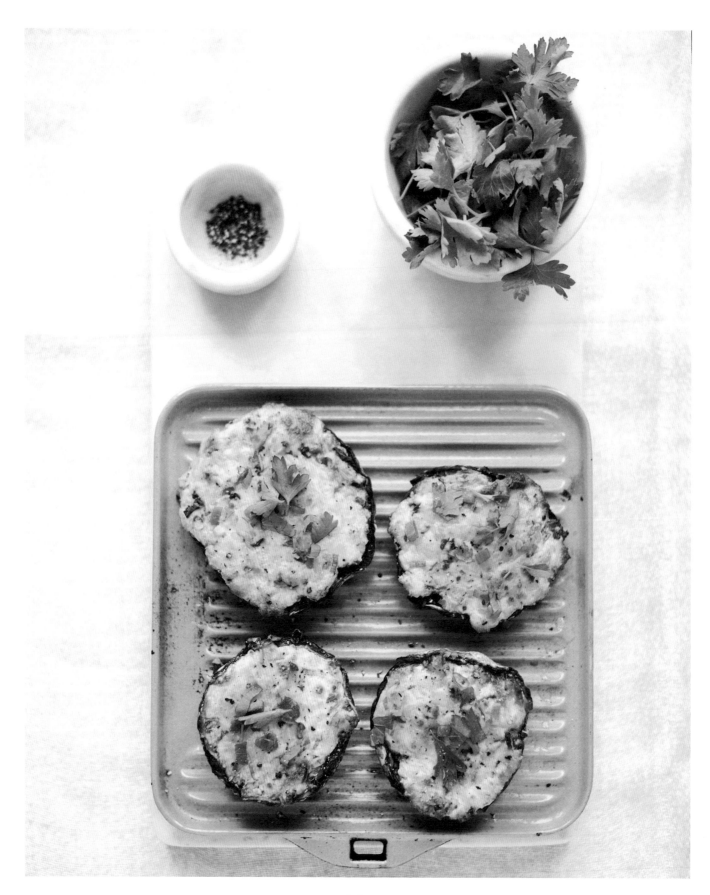

06

CHEESY PORTOBELLO MUSHROOMS

Serves 4-6

Portobello mushrooms make a satisfying meal. You can bake them with butter, and then use as a base for a hamburger or poached egg. Or you could fill them with leftovers and bake for a satisfying meal.

INGREDIENTS

- 6 Portobello mushrooms
- 125g Cheddar, finely grated
- 40g blue cheese, crumbled
- 100g cream cheese
- 1 tbsp cream or sour cream
- 3 spring onions
- Salt
- Ground pepper

METHOD

1. Preheat oven to 180°C.
2. Remove the stalks from the mushrooms and place the upturned tops in a baking dish.
3. Combine the Cheddar, blue cheese, cream cheese and cream; stir well to mix.
4. Chop the stalks and spring onions finely and add to cheese mixture.
5. Divide the mixture between the 6 mushrooms and spread out to cover the top of each.
6. Bake at 180°C for 15 minutes or until the tops are bubbling and golden.

07

CHICKEN LIVER SALAD

Serves 2

Chicken livers are so versatile. Not only are they packed with nutrition, they are also very affordable. Cook more than is needed, and use the extra for other dishes. We recommend cooking at least 500g of liver.

INGREDIENTS

- 100g chicken livers
- 1 tbsp olive oil
- 300g baby spinach or other salad leaves
- 1 avocado
- 2 spring onions, chopped
- Creamy Salad Dressing (recipe on p214)
- Parmesan shavings (optional)
- Salt and pepper

METHOD

1. Toss the chicken livers in olive oil and season them with salt and pepper. Roast at 180°C for 20-25 minutes until cooked through.
2. Alternatively, you can fry them in a pan; be careful not to break them into pieces.
3. Arrange your salad leaves on two plates, then add half an avocado to each plate and a chopped spring onion.
4. Slice the chicken livers and arrange on top of each salad.
5. Dress with Creamy Salad Dressing.
6. Top with shaved Parmesan.

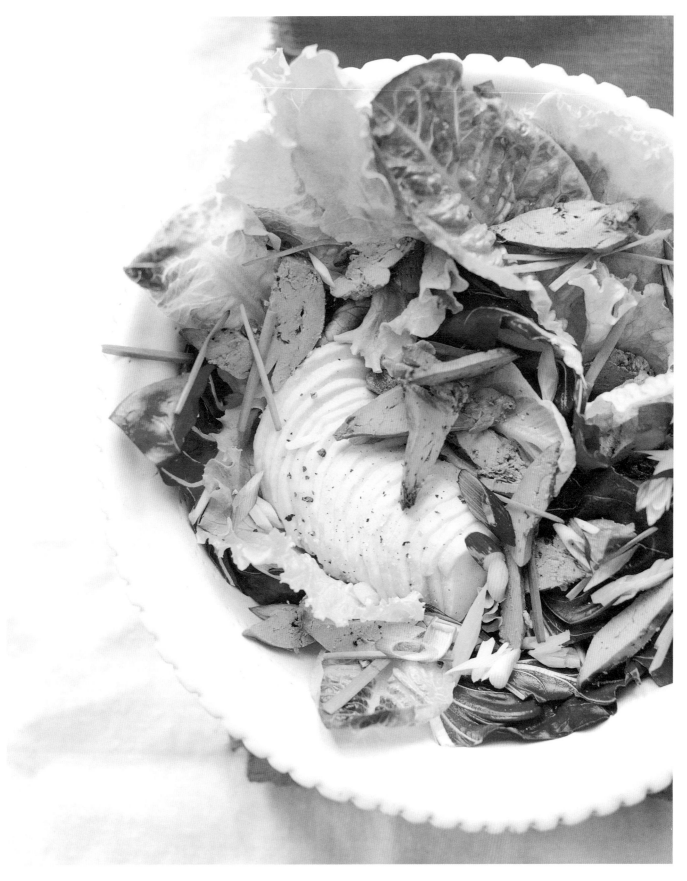

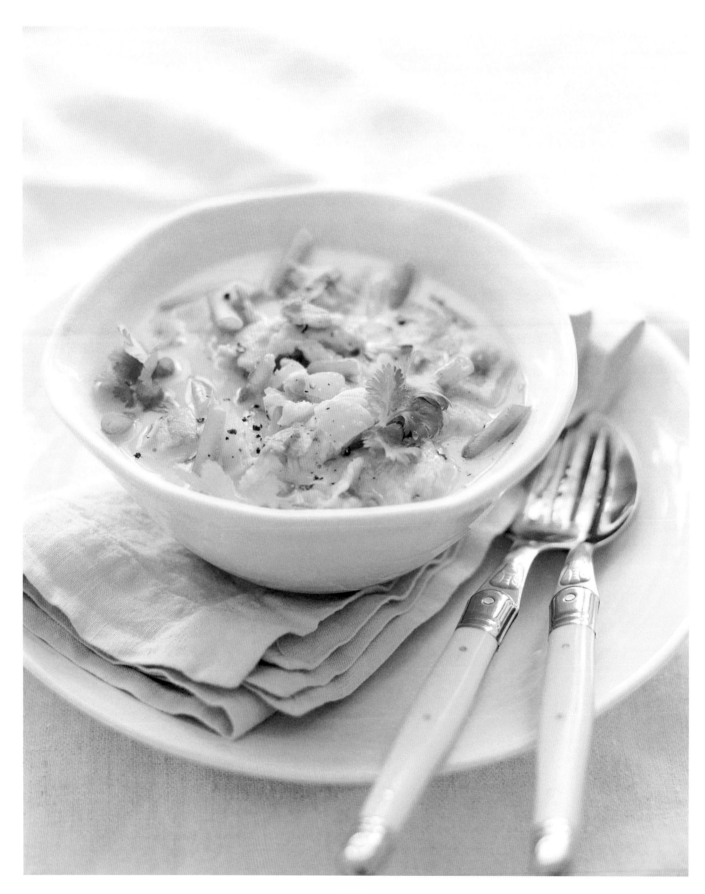

08

COCONUT THAI GREEN CHICKEN CURRY

Serves 6-8

This simple take on a Thai curry is flavoursome and easy to make. Serve with a side of vegetables, or enjoy as is as a soup. This recipe may be halved.

INGREDIENTS

- 2 medium onions, diced
- 1½ tsp fresh ginger, grated
- 8 chicken breasts (1½kg)
- 1 lime, freshly squeezed
- 2 tbsp coconut oil
- 1 garlic clove, crushed
- 800ml coconut milk
- ½-1½ tsp green curry paste (to your taste)
- Fresh coriander, handful
- 200g fresh baby green beans
- Salt and pepper
- Optional: 6 rashers bacon

METHOD

1. Finely chop the onions and grate the ginger. You could use a food processor.
2. Dice the chicken breasts into bite-sized pieces or strips. Sprinkle with black pepper and salt and a squeeze of the lime.
3. Add coconut oil to a wok on medium heat, add the chicken and cook until the meat is white.
4. Set aside.
5. In a separate pan, add the green curry paste, chopped onion, garlic and ginger and cook for approximately 5 minutes until the onions are translucent.
6. Add chicken, coconut milk and lime to the onion mixture.
7. Add a handful of fresh coriander.
8. Finally, add the green beans; chopped or whole.
9. Cover the wok and allow the food to simmer for 20-30 minutes on medium heat until the chicken is cooked through and tender.
10. Serve with cauliflower rice or steamed broccoli.

09

CAULIFLOWER RICE WITH ROAST VEGETABLES AND CHICKEN

Serves 6-8

The perfect one-dish dinner; you could also leave out the chicken and serve it as a side dish with any protein. This recipe will leave you with leftovers, and can be served hot or cold. Don't be concerned about spreading a small amount of honey over such a large amount of food; it is fine to use a little in this way. Make sure it's raw, and local. Include a few Orange-listed vegetables here for variety and taste. Work them into your carb count.

INGREDIENTS

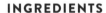

- 2 onions
- 2 peppers: 1 red, 1 yellow
- 2 medium carrots
- 1 medium sweet potato
- 4 courgettes
- 20 green beans, topped and tailed and cut in half
- 3 tbsp olive oil
- 1 tsp chilli flakes
- 1 medium cauliflower, grated or popped into the food processor
- 2 tbsp coconut oil
- 100g baby spinach, shredded
- Salt and pepper to season
- 800g cooked chicken, shredded

DRESSING

- 125ml avocado oil
- 70ml white wine vinegar
- 2 tbsp xylitol
- 2 tsp honey
- Salt and pepper to taste
- Pinch of ginger powder

METHOD

1. Cut the onions, peppers, carrots, sweet potato and courgettes into bite-sized chunks for roasting. Add the green beans, toss in the olive oil, add chilli flakes and season with salt and pepper.
2. Roast at 200°C until tender; some caramelisation on the vegetables adds to the flavour.
3. While the vegetables are roasting, fry the cauli-rice in the coconut oil, until just tender. Do not overcook.
4. Put the cauli-rice on a serving platter.
5. As the roast vegetables come out of the oven, stir in the baby spinach. It will wilt easily.
6. Now plate the roast vegetables on top of the cauli-rice. Top this with shredded chicken.
7. Whisk together the dressing ingredients, taste and adjust seasoning accordingly.
8. Drizzle the dressing over the dish, or serve on the side.

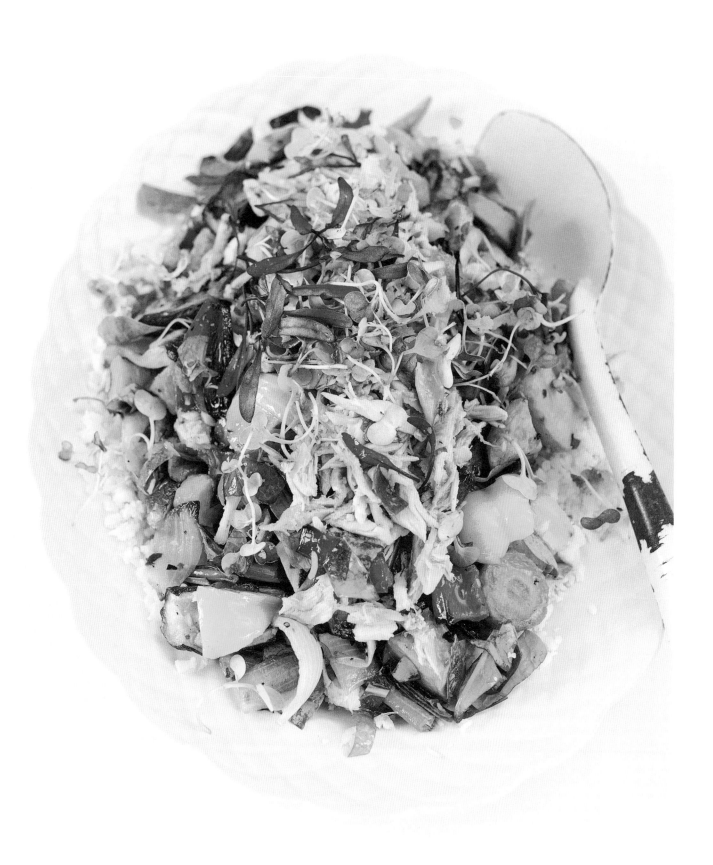

10

CORONATION CHICKEN

Serves 4-6

Serve this with a salad, with toasted almond flakes on the side.

INGREDIENTS

- 150ml Homemade Mayonnaise (see recipe p216)
- 1 tsp curry powder
- 2 tsp freshly squeezed lemon juice
- Onion chutney
- 500g cooked chicken, diced
- Salt to taste

METHOD

1. Combine the mayonnaise, curry powder, lemon juice and onion chutney. Add salt to taste.
2. Stir in the diced chicken.

Onion chutney

INGREDIENTS

- 1 tbsp coconut oil
- 2 onions, thinly sliced
- 1 tbsp xylitol
- 2 tbsp wine vinegar
- 2 tbsp balsamic vinegar

METHOD

1. Fry the onions in the coconut oil until translucent.
2. Add xylitol and vinegar to the onions and simmer for about 10 minutes until the liquid seems to disappear.
3. Allow the chutney to cool before you use it.

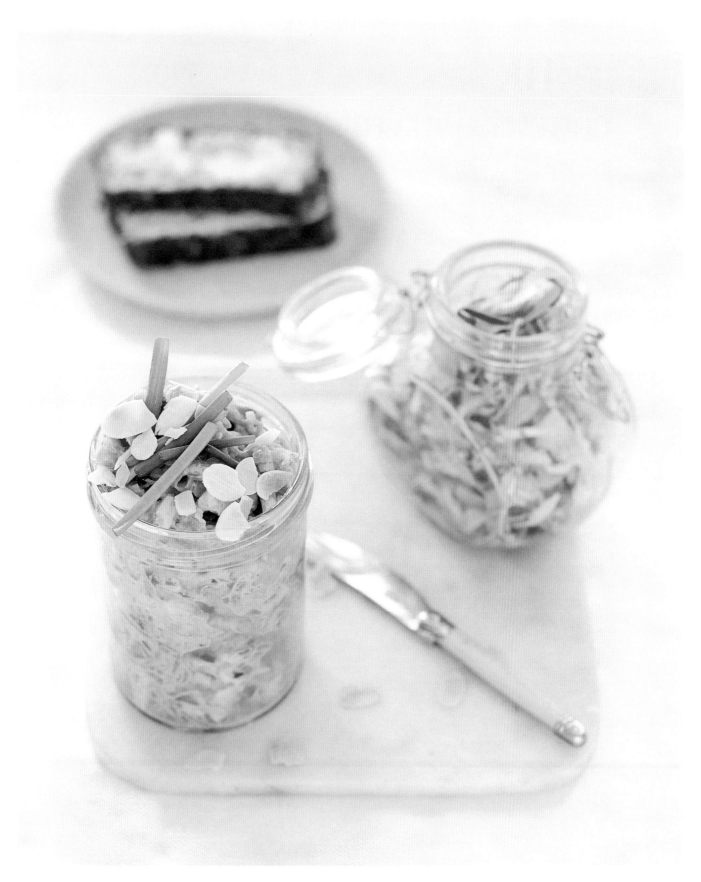

11

CREAMY TOMATO CHICKEN
Serves 4

Use the Versatile Tomato Sauce recipe and some full fat plain yoghurt to create this simple, yet divine chicken dish.

INGREDIENTS

- 4 chicken breasts on the bone, butterflied (about 1kg) (you can use boneless chicken breast, but tenderise with a meat mallet before seasoning)
- 1 lemon
- 4 sprigs of rosemary
- 2½ tsp mixed dried herbs
- 2 medium onions, quartered
- Salt and pepper
- 250ml Versatile Tomato Sauce (recipe p219)
- 250ml full fat plain yoghurt
- 1 handful fresh coriander

METHOD

1. Preheat oven to 180°C.
2. Mix yoghurt and tomato sauce together in a bowl.
3. Season chicken liberally with salt and pepper and a squeeze of fresh lemon.
4. Cut the onions into quarters.
5. Lay the chicken into an ovenproof dish, add 4 sprigs of rosemary and nestle the onion quarters between the chicken breasts. Sprinkle with dried herbs.
6. Cover the chicken with the yoghurt and tomato sauce mixture.
7. Bake for 40 minutes until the chicken is moist and cooked through.
8. Garnish with fresh coriander. Serve with vegetables or fresh salad.

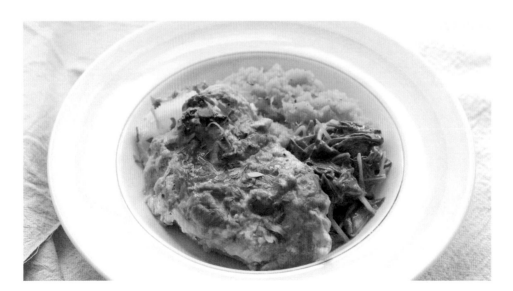

12

CABBAGE CARBONARA

Serves 4

This is a delicious way to serve cabbage – bacon, cabbage and cream – it doesn't get better than this.

INGREDIENTS

- 12 slices of streaky bacon, diced
- 700g cabbage, shredded
- 2 cloves garlic, crushed
- 120ml double cream
- 2 egg yolks
- Salt and pepper
- Shaved Parmesan cheese

METHOD

1. Fry bacon until all the fat is rendered.
2. Remove the cooked bacon and place onto a plate.
3. Sauté the cabbage in the bacon fat until it is tender but not mushy – about 5 minutes.
4. Add the garlic and the cream (reserve 2 tsp for the eggs) and simmer till the mixture thickens.
5. Whisk the egg yolks with the reserved cream.
6. Remove the dish from the heat, add the egg yolk mixture and bacon, stir well.
7. Season with salt and pepper.
8. Top with shavings of Parmesan and serve.

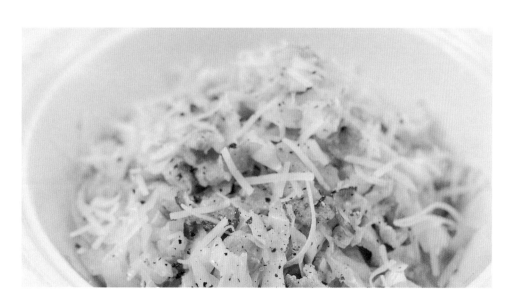

13

AUBERGINE PARMIGIANA

Serves 6

A favourite vegetarian dish. It takes a lot of work, but it's completely worth the effort as the flavours are simply sublime. Make it with the aubergines peeled or unpeeled, your choice.

INGREDIENTS

- 1½kg aubergines, peeled and sliced lengthways
- Fine rock salt, black pepper to season
- 2 tbsp extra virgin olive oil
- 3 cloves of garlic, crushed
- 800g quality tinned tomatoes without sugar
- 100ml vinegar or 120ml red wine
- 2 tsp xylitol
- ½ tsp dried oregano (preferably fresh)
- 75g butter or 75ml coconut oil to fry
- 200g mozzarella, grated
- 125g Parmesan, grated
- 50g desiccated coconut for crumbs
- Handful of basil leaves

METHOD

1. Sprinkle a little salt over the aubergine slices and leave in a colander over a sink to sweat and drain for 30 minutes.

TOMATO SAUCE

1. While the aubergines are sweating, heat the olive oil to a medium temperature.
2. Add the crushed garlic. Heat for a minute.
3. Add the tomatoes and vinegar (or wine). Bring to the boil, then turn down the heat to the lowest setting.
4. Add xylitol, salt, pepper and oregano and simmer for approximately 40-50 minutes with the lid off. Check and stir regularly.
5. Use a stick blender to purée the tomato sauce until smooth, and set aside.

AUBERGINE PREP

1. Preheat the oven to 180°C.
2. Rinse the aubergines well, and pat dry with kitchen paper.
3. Pour enough coconut oil into a frying pan to coat the bottom well, and put on a high heat.
4. Fry the aubergine slices until golden brown on both sides, working in batches. Add more coconut oil as needed as the aubergines soak up the coconut oil. Put the cooked slices on paper towel to drain.
5. Grease an oven dish lightly with butter, and spread the bottom with a layer of tomato sauce. Follow with a layer of tightly packed aubergine.
6. Top the aubergine with grated mozzarella and a sprinkling of Parmesan. Repeat, starting with the tomato again, then aubergine and then cheese. Finish the top layer of sauce with some Parmesan and desiccated coconut. Bake for 30 minutes, until bubbling.

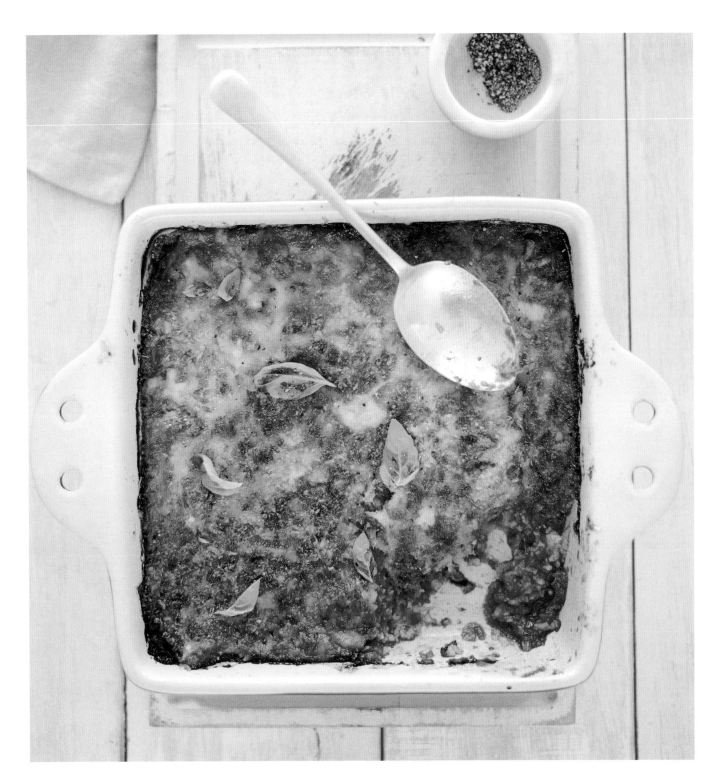

Add some basil pesto or fresh pesto after each aubergine layer and then top with cheese,
to create a Caprese Aubergine Parmigiana.

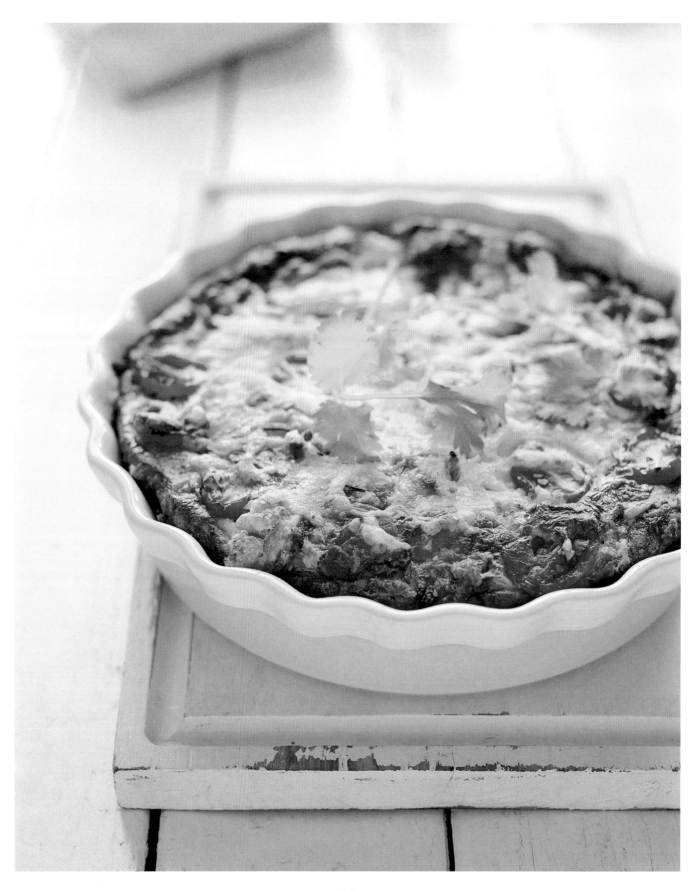

14

FARM-STYLE CRUSTLESS QUICHE

Serves 6

I simply love quiche as a meal. It's perfect for breakfast, lunch with salad and even better in a lunch box or picnic basket. It's not easy catering for everyone's tastes. A little bit of everyone's favourite things all poured into one delicious meal. Every bite is different.

INGREDIENTS

- 200g streaky bacon, diced and cooked
- 1 tbsp coconut oil
- 1 medium onion, diced
- 70g mushrooms, washed and sliced
- 5 whole eggs
- 5 egg whites
- 250ml double cream
- 1 tbsp coconut flour
- 2 spring onions, chopped
- 60g Cheddar cheese, grated
- 60g mozzarella cheese, grated
- 8 cherry tomatoes, halved
- 1 round feta cheese, crumbled
- Salt and pepper to taste
- 1 tbsp chives, diced

METHOD

1. Preheat your oven to 180°C.
2. Dice the streaky bacon and cook on medium heat in a pan. Set aside.
3. Heat coconut oil in a pan, and add onion and mushrooms and cook until tender.
4. Add bacon and combine. Set aside.
5. In a large mixing bowl, combine eggs, egg whites, cream and coconut flour and mix well.
6. Add a pinch of salt and pepper, cheese and chopped spring onions.
7. Stir the egg and cheese, and bacon mixture together in the large bowl.
8. Grease a 25cm pie plate or baking dish with coconut oil or butter.
9. Pour the quiche mixture into the baking dish and dot with the sliced cherry tomatoes. Finish off with crumbled feta.
10. Bake for approximately 45 minutes until golden brown.
11. Remove from oven and garnish with chives.

01

BROCCOLI

Serves 4

Broccoli is one of the most versatile of all vegetables, high in protein and packed with phytochemicals.

Roasted broccoli

INGREDIENTS

- 1 head of broccoli, cut into florets with stem (cut each into halves or quarters, depending on how big the piece is)
- 50ml olive oil
- Salt

METHOD

1. Put all the cut pieces in a large bowl and toss with the olive oil.
2. Place in a single layer on a baking sheet; you may want to use two sheets to make sure that the broccoli has space.
3. Season with salt.
4. Bake at 180°C for 15-25 minutes, until the stems are tender and the florets start to go crispy. Keep checking so that you don't burn the broccoli.

VARIATION

1. Toss the chopped florets with an egg seasoned with salt and pepper until they are well coated. Add 100g grated Parmesan and toss to cover.
2. Spread out on a well-greased baking tray. Bake at 200°C for 10-15 minutes. Again, you will need to check and adjust according to your oven.

Broccoli with nuts

INGREDIENTS

- 2 tbsp olive oil
- 1 clove garlic, crushed
- 85g macadamia nuts or flaked almonds
- 250g broccoli, chopped into small florets.

METHOD

1. Heat olive oil, add garlic and nuts.
2. Fry until nuts are lightly golden.
3. Add broccoli and stir-fry until just tender.

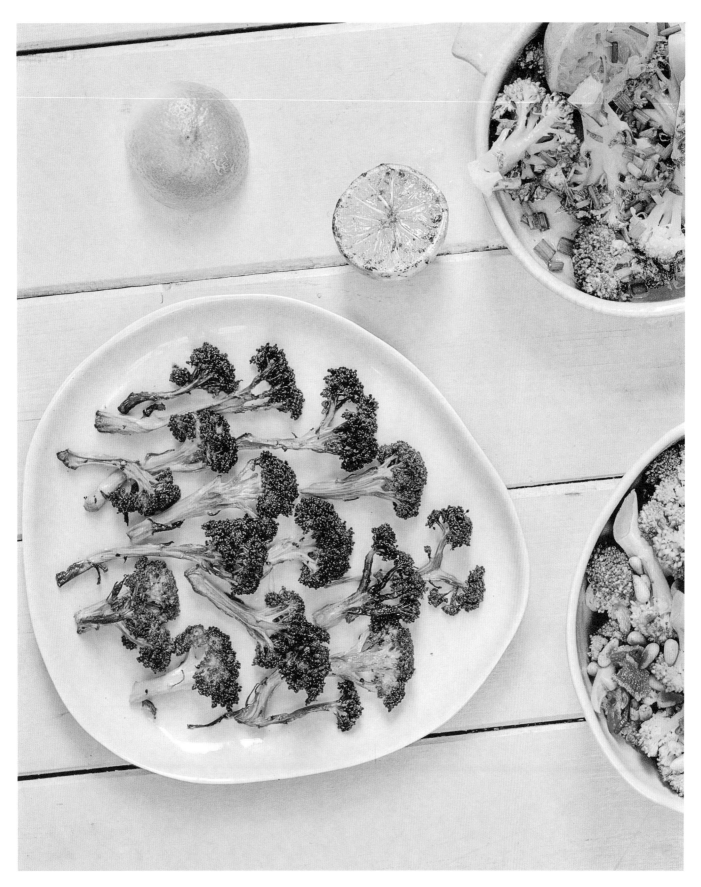

Broccoli with bacon and pine nuts

INGREDIENTS

- 2 tbsp coconut oil
- 2 rashers bacon, finely sliced
- 250g broccoli, cut into florets
- 2 tbsp pine nuts, toasted
- 2 tbsp chives, chopped

METHOD

1. Heat coconut oil, add bacon.
2. Once cooked, add broccoli florets, fry until just tender.
3. Add toasted pine nuts and chopped chives.

Broccoli with mustard butter

INGREDIENTS

- 250g broccoli, cut into florets
- 75g butter
- 2 tbsp Dijon mustard
- Ground black pepper

METHOD

1. Steam broccoli florets until just tender.
2. Combine softened butter with Dijon mustard, along with some ground black pepper. Serve over hot broccoli.
3. If you are having a dinner party, pipe rosettes of mustard butter onto grease-proof paper and let it set in the fridge. You can then put a rosette onto the broccoli on each plate.

Broccoli dressed with olive oil and lemon

INGREDIENTS

- 250g broccoli, cut into florets
- 2 tbsp olive oil
- 1 tbsp lemon juice
- Salt and ground black pepper
- Chilli flakes (optional)

METHOD

1. Steam broccoli until just tender.
2. Combine olive oil, lemon juice, salt and ground black pepper (add some chilli flakes if you wish).
3. Toss with the hot broccoli and serve.

Buttered broccoli

INGREDIENTS

- 50g butter
- 250g broccoli, cut into florets
- 4 tbsp fresh herbs, chopped (chives, parsley, flat leaf parsley, coriander and basil are all good, either individually or in combination)

METHOD

1. Heat butter in a pan and add broccoli florets.
2. Cover and cook over medium heat until tender.
3. Stir through chopped herbs.

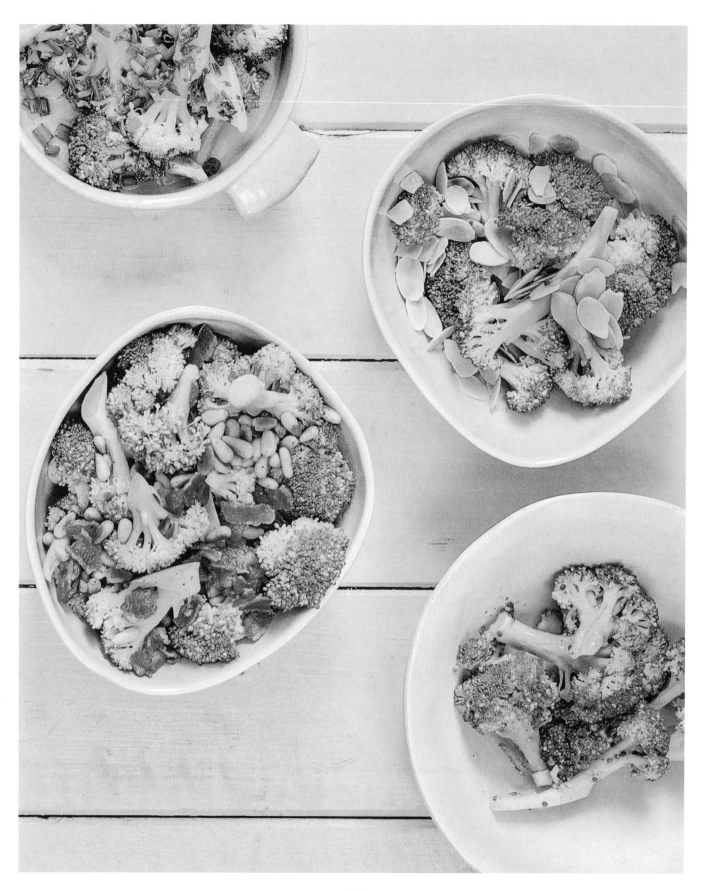

02

CABBAGE

Serves 4-6

Cabbage is a versatile and tasty vegetable that we simply love. Here are some delightful and simple recipes to turn this vegetable into your home favourite.

Sautéed cabbage

This is a fantastic option to serve with curry or stew. It can also be used as an alternative to spaghetti and served with a pasta-like sauce. If you cook extra, you can use it in breakfast the following day.

INGREDIENTS

- 50g of butter, lard or tallow
- ½ small or ¼ large cabbage, shredded
- Salt and pepper

METHOD

1. Melt the butter.
2. Add the cabbage and sauté until tender.
3. Season with salt and pepper.

Baked or barbecued baby cabbage

INGREDIENTS

- 2 baby cabbages
- 50g butter, softened
- Salt and pepper
- Chilli flakes
- Streaky bacon

METHOD

1. Split the cabbages into four without going through the stalk.
2. Smear the inside of each cabbage with butter.
3. Season with salt and pepper and chilli flakes.
4. Wrap a rasher of streaky bacon through the split (this can be left out if you don't eat bacon).
5. Wrap each cabbage individually in aluminium foil.
6. To barbecue, place on the coals, turn regularly, and cook for about 40 minutes. Or bake it at 180°C for 45 minutes.

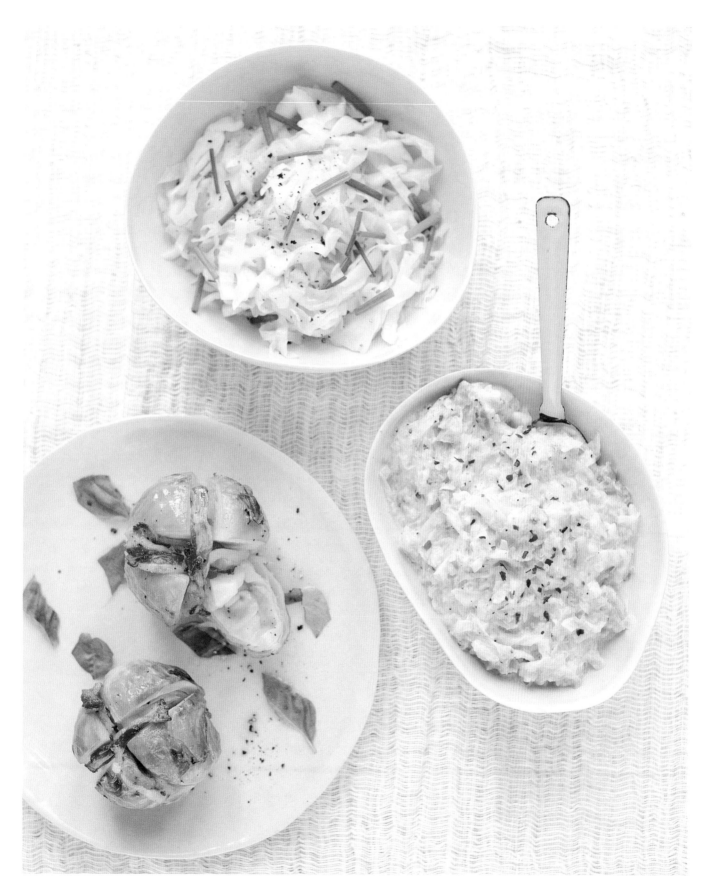

Decadent creamy cabbage

This cooks for a long time; the longer the better, so make extra. Leftovers are wonderful warmed in a pan; make holes in the mixture and break in your eggs so that they cook with the cabbage around them.

INGREDIENTS

- 100g lard or butter
- 1 onion, sliced
- 4 rashers of bacon, chopped (optional)
- ½ cabbage, shredded
- 60ml water
- Salt, ground pepper, and chilli flakes (optional)
- 250ml cream

METHOD

1. Melt the lard or butter and fry the onion and bacon if you are using it.
2. Add cabbage and make sure it is coated in the lard.
3. Add water, turn down the heat, put the lid on the pan and cook until very soft (20-30 minutes or more, you may have to add extra water).
4. Once the cabbage is soft, remove the lid and allow the excess water to cook off.
5. Season with salt, ground pepper and chilli flakes.
6. Add cream and stir, bring to a simmer and allow it to thicken.

Coleslaw (with a difference)

INGREDIENTS

- ½ green cabbage, finely shredded
- 3 carrots, coarsely grated
- 6 radishes, coarsely grated
- 1 red pepper, chopped
- 4 spring onions, sliced
- small bunch flat leaf parsley, chopped
- 250ml Homemade Mayonnaise (see p218)
- Salt and pepper to season

METHOD

Add mayonnaise to the rest of the ingredients, season with salt and ground pepper and toss until well combined.

TIP

For a special event, use half green cabbage and half red cabbage for visual appeal. You could also ribbon your carrots and thinly slice your radishes.

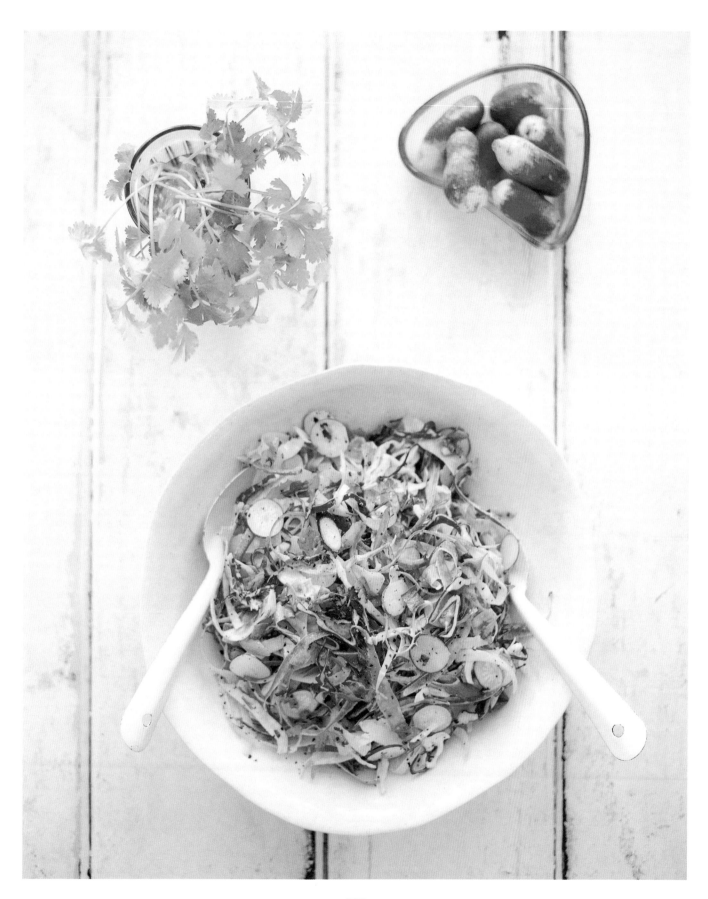

03

BEST CAULIFLOWER EVER Serves 6-8

The addition of sour cream, garlic and mushrooms makes this a cauliflower dish even little Timmy will gladly eat.

INGREDIENTS

- 1 head of cauliflower, cut into small florets
- 1 onion, chopped
- 1 red pepper, chopped
- 2 cloves garlic, crushed
- 250g mushrooms, sliced
- 100g bacon (optional)
- 50g butter
- 250ml sour cream
- 250g of cream cheese
- Seasoning
- 120g cheese, grated

METHOD

1. Steam the cauliflower until just tender, then put it into a greased ovenproof dish.
2. In a pan, fry the onion, pepper, garlic, mushrooms and bacon (if you are using it) and season with salt and pepper while cooking. If you like a bit of heat, you can add some chilli flakes.
3. Toss the fried mixture through the cauliflower.
4. Now mix the cream cheese and sour cream together and spread it evenly over the top (on cooking it will spread into the cauliflower).
5. Top the mixture with grated cheese and bake at 180°C for 20 minutes until the cheese is melted and the dish is piping hot.

TIP

For extra decadence, you can add a cup of cheese into the sour cream and cream cheese mix. You can also add other protein and turn this into a meal. Leftover shredded chicken works very well.

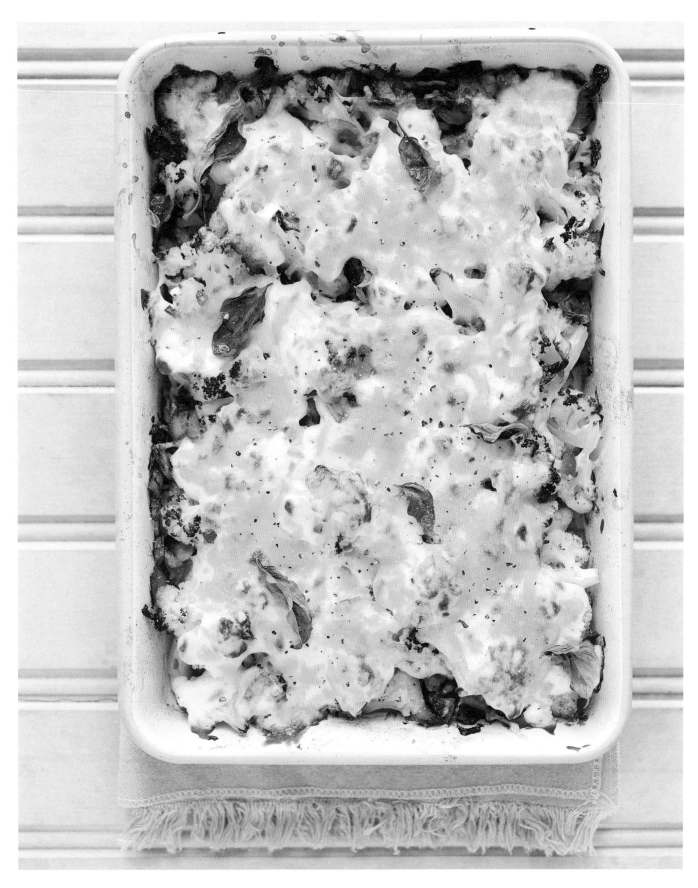

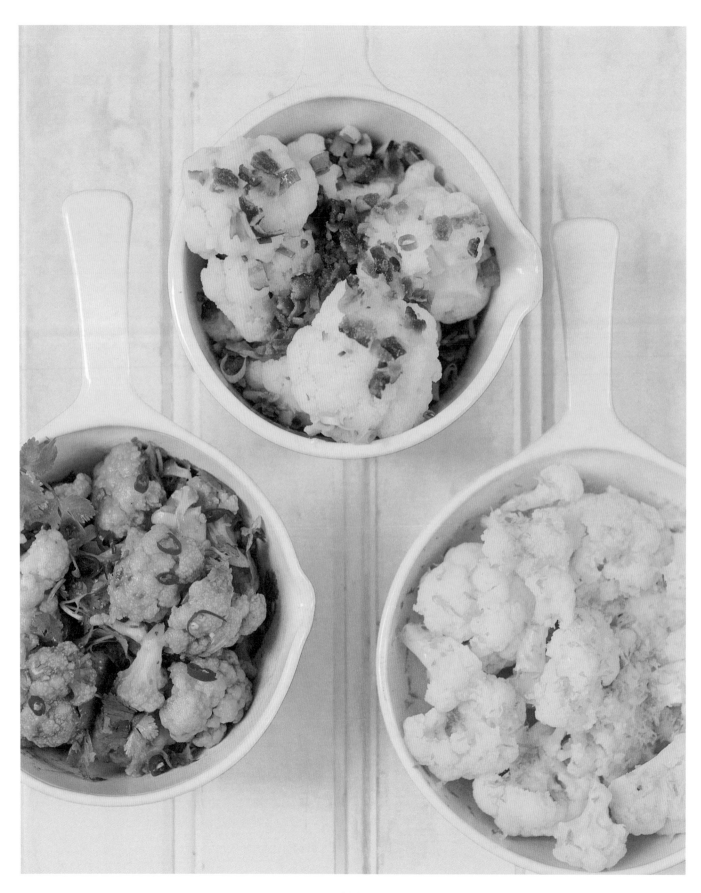

04

OPTIONS FOR STEAMED CAULIFLOWER

Here are some options for cauliflower when you are really at a loss. Cut 400g of cauliflower into small florets, steam until just tender, and use one of these below options.

CHILLI

In a large bowl combine:

- 50g butter, melted
- 1 tbsp tomato paste
- 2 tbsp coriander, chopped
- ½ tsp chilli powder

Add the cooked cauliflower, toss and serve hot.

LIME OR LEMON

In a large bowl combine:

- 50g butter, melted
- 1 tbsp lime or lemon juice
- 1 tsp rind, finely grated
- 1 clove garlic, crushed
- 1 tsp honey

Add the cooked cauliflower, toss and serve hot.

BACON

- 4 rashers bacon, chopped
- 15g butter
- 2 spring onions, finely sliced

Fry the bacon in the butter until crispy, then toss the butter and bacon with the cauliflower. Add the sliced spring onions and stir to combine. Serve hot.

05

PUMPKIN

As pumpkin is so versatile, it is a good idea to bake more than you need. The leftovers can be used in other recipes. It's Orange list, but should you want to make a soup for the family members who are Paleo or not very rigid, these are lovely recipes.

Baked pumpkin

INGREDIENTS

- Several large pieces of pumpkin
- Melted butter
- Olive oil

METHOD

1. Place the pumpkin pieces into a baking dish. Brush liberally with a mixture of melted butter and olive oil.
2. The amount you need will depend on how much pumpkin you have – be generous.
3. Bake at 180°C for 40 minutes, or until the pumpkin is golden and cooked through.
4. Serve this as a vegetable accompaniment to a meat meal.

Pumpkin salad

INGREDIENTS

- 180g baked pumpkin, cubed
- 100g salad leaves; rocket is particularly good
- 100g feta
- ¼ red onion, thinly sliced

Put all the ingredients into a large serving bowl.

DRESSING

- 100ml olive oil
- 2 tbsp lemon juice
- Salt and ground pepper

METHOD

1. Whisk the ingredients together and drizzle over the salad.
2. To turn it into a main meal, add some crispy bacon or Prosciutto to the top of the salad once you have added the dressing.

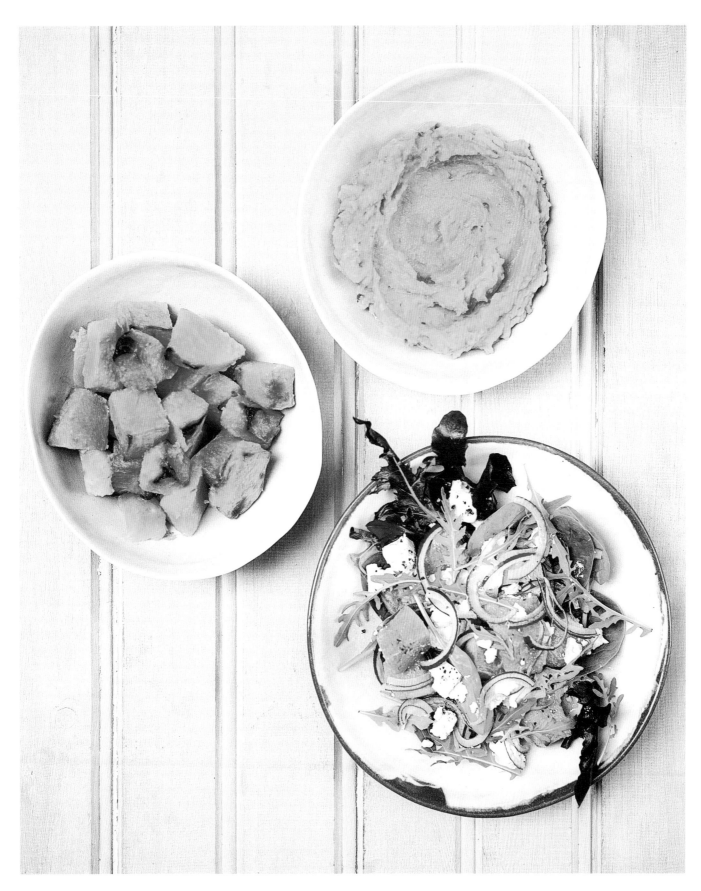

Pumpkin purée

INGREDIENTS

- 500g pumpkin, steamed
- 50g butter
- Pinch of ground nutmeg
- Salt and pepper to taste

METHOD

1. Mash the steamed pumpkin with a potato masher.
2. Add the butter and nutmeg and season with salt and pepper.

Pumpkin soup

INGREDIENTS

- 360g of mashed pumpkin
- 50g butter
- 125ml chicken broth
- 60ml full cream milk
- 125ml cream
- Salt and pepper to taste

METHOD

1. Put all ingredients except cream into a food processor and blend until smooth.
2. Transfer to a pot and stir in the cream and heat gently.
3. Season to taste.
4. Alternatively, heat all ingredients in a pot and use a stick blender.

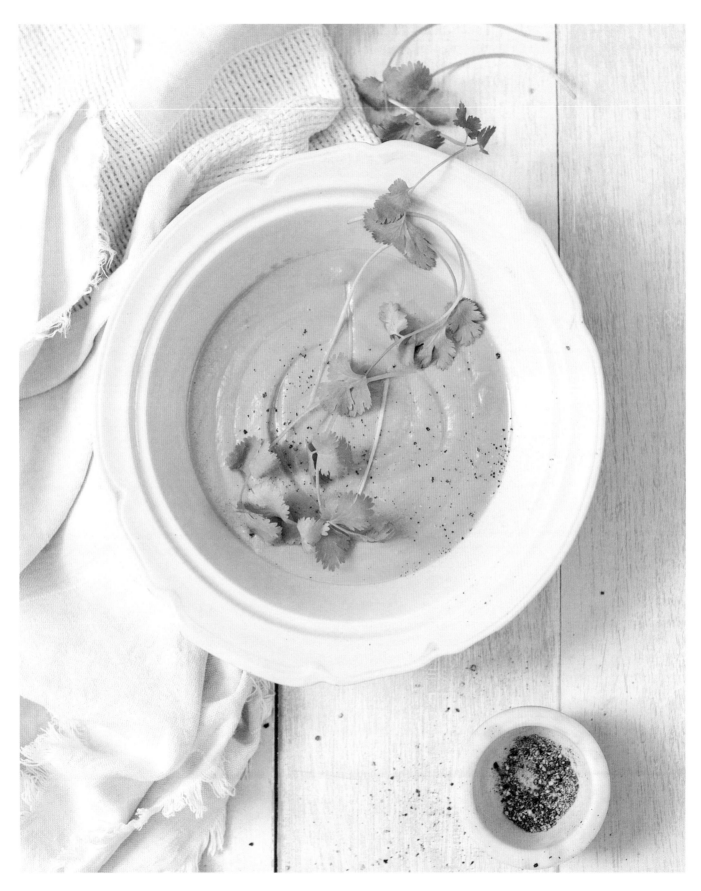

06

CHICKEN BROTH

Serves 4

Make this broth regularly and freeze into 500ml portions as you can use this as a stock for many recipes.

INGREDIENTS

- Saved chicken bones or a roasting chicken
- ½ tsp salt
- 6 peppercorns
- 1 onion
- 2 stems of celery with leaves
- 2 medium carrots
- 1 tbsp apple cider vinegar
- A stem of fresh rosemary or thyme (or herbs of your choice)

METHOD

1. Roast a whole chicken in a slow cooker or in a crock-pot until done. Remove all the skin and add it to your stockpot. Strip the bones and save the meat for another recipe. Add the bones to your stockpot. If using saved carcasses, place them in the pot.
2. Roughly chop all your other ingredients and add to your pot. Now add water to cover the bones.
3. Simmer for 8 hours. Strain the liquid and discard the bones, vegetables, peppercorns and herbs.
4. Immediately freeze in serving sizes for later use.

TIP

- Save the carcasses of your chickens and freeze them. When you have a few, use them to make broth.
- You can make bone broth in a slow cooker.
- Do not boil rapidly as it will spoil the taste of your broth.

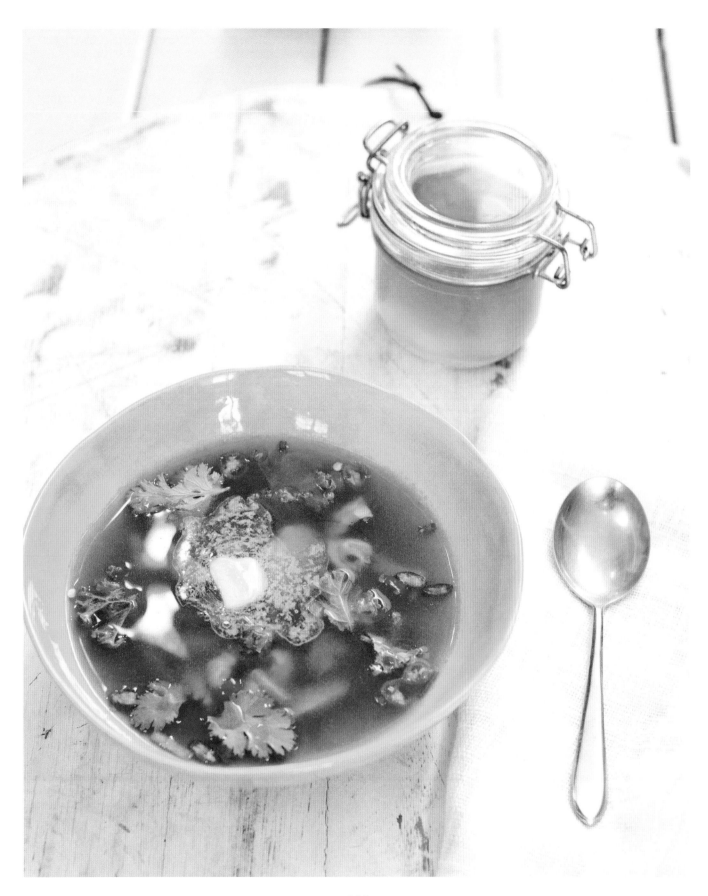

07

TABOULI

Serves 4-6

This is a perfect salad to make hours before you need it. Tabouli tastes much better once the flavours have had time to meld. It can, however, be eaten straight away. Leftovers will be perfect for a lunch, with some added protein.

INGREDIENTS

METHOD

- 50ml olive or coconut oil
- 200g cauli-rice
- 2 large tomatoes, chopped
- 4 spring onions, chopped
- 1 yellow pepper, finely chopped
- 60g flat-leaf parsley, chopped
- 10g mint, chopped
- Salt and ground pepper

1. Heat the oil in a saucepan and fry the cauli-rice until just cooked. The grains must still easily separate. Allow it to cool.
2. Combine all the ingredients in a large bowl.
3. Season with salt and ground pepper.
4. Whisk together the dressing ingredients and add to the salad.
5. Allow the flavours to mingle.

DRESSING

- 120ml olive oil
- 60ml lemon juice
- 1 clove garlic, crushed

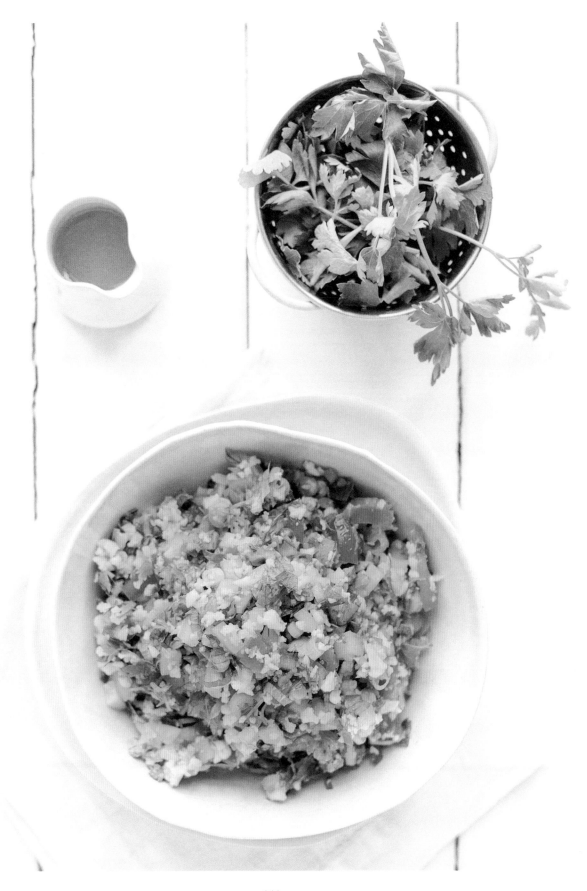

01

CREAMY SALAD DRESSING Makes 200ml

Although this dressing is delicious freshly made, if you can make it in advance the flavours will have time to develop. Any extra can be stored in the fridge for a week. You can also double the recipe as it stores well.

INGREDIENTS

- 1 tsp xylitol
- 1 tsp mixed herbs
- 1 clove garlic, crushed
- 150ml olive, avocado or macadamia nut oil
- 25ml wine vinegar
- 1 egg
- Salt and ground pepper to taste

METHOD

Put all ingredients in a blender, or use a stick blender to mix.

VARIATION

You can alter the dressing by adding any of the following to the ingredients. Either blend them with the rest of the ingredients or add them after blending.

1. Chilli flakes
2. Mustard powder
3. Chopped parsley
4. Spring onions
5. Chopped coriander
6. Chopped basil
7. Fresh rosemary

The photograph is of the Creamy Salad Dressing made with fresh basil which turns it a delightful shade of green.

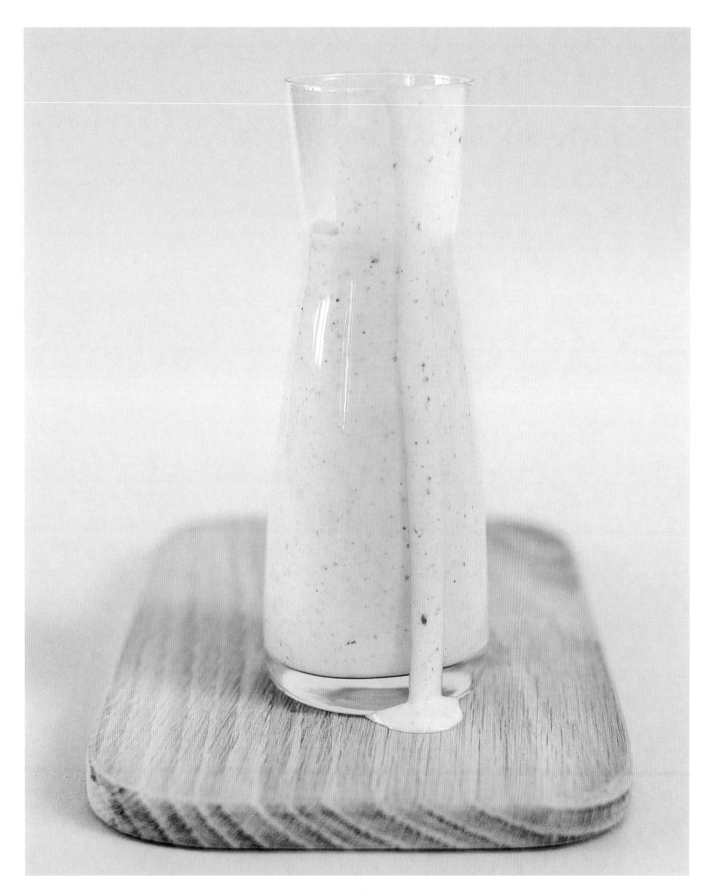

02

LIQUIDISER HOLLANDAISE

Makes 200ml

The easiest Hollandaise ever, you can even make it in a smoothie machine. Once you have this mastered, there are lots of recipes that call for Hollandaise sauce.

INGREDIENTS

- 1 tbsp white wine vinegar
- 1 tbsp lemon juice
- 3 egg yolks
- 150g butter, melted
- Salt and pepper

METHOD

1. Put the wine vinegar and lemon juice in a saucepan and bring to the boil.
2. Put the egg yolks and a grind of salt in the liquidiser and start blending.
3. With the liquidiser still running, pour in the hot liquid in a steady stream.
4. Slowly add the melted butter, with the liquidiser still running. Now adjust your seasoning.

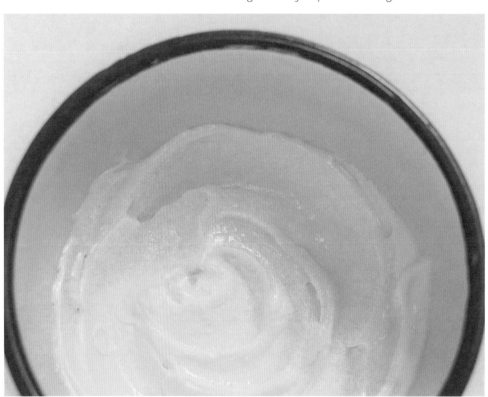

03

CREAMY MUSHROOM SAUCE Makes 200ml

This versatile sauce is delicious served with steak, or over vegetables.

INGREDIENTS

- 250g button mushrooms, chopped
- 30g butter
- 200ml cream
- 125g Cheddar cheese, grated
- Salt and pepper

METHOD

1. Fry mushrooms in butter until cooked and brown.
2. Add cream and slowly bring to the boil.
3. Once it comes to the boil, take your pot off the heat and stir in the cheese, which will melt and thicken your sauce.
4. Season with salt and pepper.

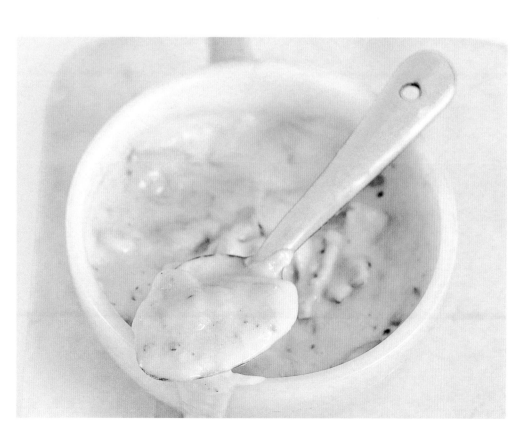

04

HOMEMADE MAYONNAISE

Makes 250ml

This mayonnaise is made with a stick blender. It is best made in the container that you will store it in; a 500ml straight-sided glass jar is perfect.

INGREDIENTS

- 1 egg
- 2 tsp lemon juice
- 2 tsp white or apple cider vinegar
- Salt and ground pepper
- 250ml of avocado oil (or macadamia or olive oil)

METHOD

1. In a jar, layer the ingredients in order so that the egg will be at the bottom and the oil will be poured on last.
2. Put your stick blender to the bottom of the jar and blend. Once the mixture starts turning white and thick, you can slowly move the blender up in the jar. The whole process takes 30 seconds.

VARIATION

This is the basic recipe, but you can vary it by adding:

- Chilli flakes
- 2 tsp Dijon mustard
- Fresh parsley, chopped
- Fresh basil, chopped

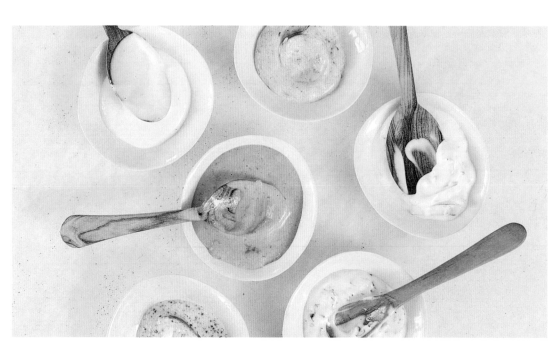

05

VERSATILE TOMATO SAUCE

Makes about a litre

Changing your family from using store-bought sauces can be a challenge at first, but you can win them over with this tomato sauce which you can use as a base for almost every tomato-based dish in your home. Add it to mince, use it to add tang to a ratatouille or convert it to a relish with ease. Bottle it and store in the fridge for frequent use.

INGREDIENTS

- 410g tomato purée
- 410g tin whole tomatoes, with no preservatives, only tomato and salt
- 60ml apple cider vinegar
- ½ tsp black pepper
- 2 tsp salt
- ½ tsp crushed garlic
- 4 tbsp xylitol
- ½ tsp psyllium husk
- 1 tsp fresh or ½ tsp dried oregano

METHOD

1. Place all the ingredients except the psyllium husk into a heavy pan on medium heat. Allow to gently simmer and reduce for 15-20 minutes.
2. Remove from heat, and stir in the psyllium husk, a sprinkle at a time. Allow to cool, then blitz with a stick blender till smooth or leave chunky and store in a glass jar in the fridge.

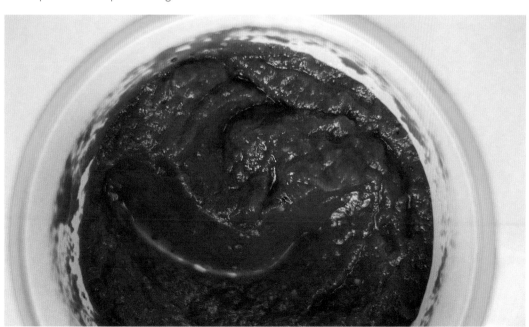

06

SWEET RED PEPPER CHILLI RELISH

Makes about a litre

If you are not a fan of chilli, leave it out. You can always add more if you want it hotter. This makes a large quantity, is fantastic to bottle and is delicious with meat and vegetables. This recipe can be halved if preferred.

INGREDIENTS

- 4 large onions
- 8 red peppers
- 5 tomatoes
- 100ml coconut oil
- 3 red chillies (or according to taste)
- 3 cloves garlic, crushed
- 60g xylitol
- 125ml wine vinegar
- Salt and pepper to taste

METHOD

1. Chop the onions, red peppers and tomatoes. A food processor makes this job very easy, but it can also be done by hand.
2. In a large pot, melt the coconut oil, add the chopped vegetables and start to heat the mixture.
3. Cut the chillies in half and add them to the mixture. If you like pieces of chilli in your relish, you can slice them. Halved chillies give flavour and can be removed after cooking.
4. Add garlic to the mixture.
5. Now add the xylitol and vinegar and bring the mixture to a simmer. Simmer for 2 hours with the lid on the pot.
6. Remove the pot lid and simmer until the mixture reduces to a nice thick syrupy sauce, this will take at least 1 hour and sometimes even longer. Check the relish frequently.
7. Once you are happy with the consistency, add salt and pepper to taste. At this point, you may remove the chillies.
8. You now have two options: you can blend the mixture to make a sweet chilli sauce, or cool it and bottle it.

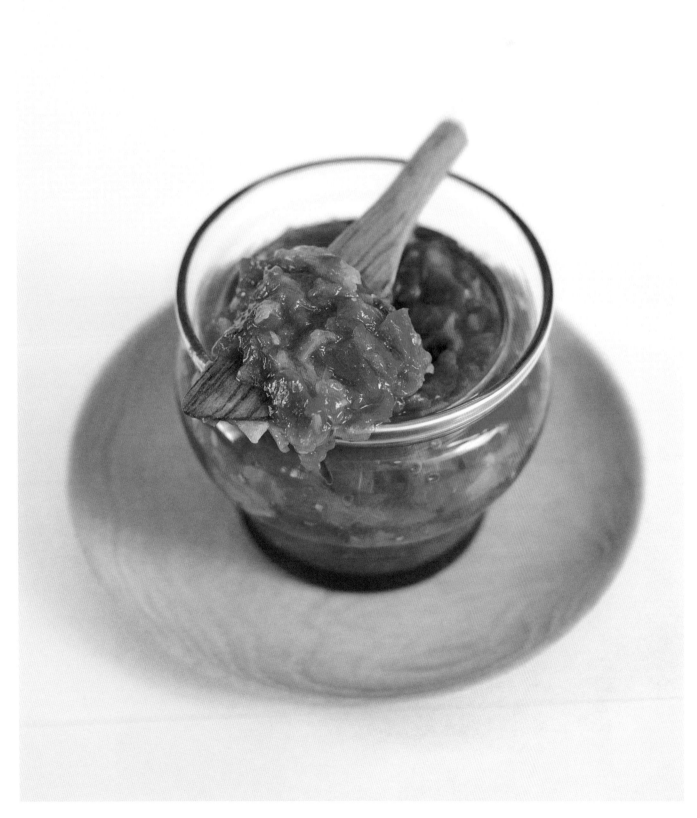

01

OLIVE AND ROSEMARY SEED CRACKERS

Makes around 24

Seed crackers are a great snack item that can be prepared in advance and keep and travel well. Perfect for a snack, light lunch or lunch box.

INGREDIENTS

- 210g sunflower seeds
- 90g flax seeds
- 30g sesame seeds
- 10g psyllium husk
- ¼ tsp or pinch Himalayan rock salt
- 40g dried olives, chopped
- 1 tbsp fresh rosemary, chopped
- 500ml water

Use a silicone mat – approx. 48 x 36cm

METHOD

1. Preheat oven to 160°C.
2. Measure out all the above ingredients into a large bowl.
3. Add water and mix with wooden spoon until blended.
4. Set aside for 10 minutes until the mixture is gooey and gummy.
5. Line your baking tray with a silicone mat.
6. Spread mixture as thinly as possible, making sure there are no holes or gaps in the spread.
7. Bake for 50 minutes, then remove the tray from the oven.
8. Score the crackers into the desired shapes.
9. Return the tray to the oven.
10. Bake for a further 30 minutes.
11. Enjoy with butter, nut butter or homemade dips.

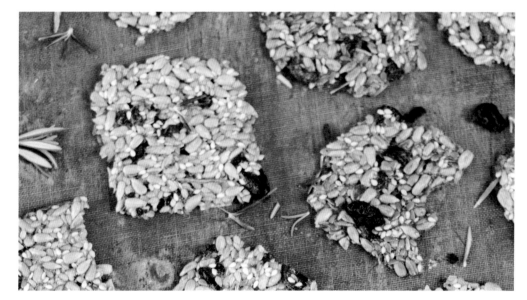

02

CHEESY
SEED BISCUITS

Makes 16-20

Make these for a special occasion. They are delicious with pâtés, pestos or cheese, or as part of a finger food lunch.

INGREDIENTS

- 250g mozzarella, grated
- 100g Parmesan
- 130g mixed seeds of your choice
- 2 egg whites
- Salt
- Ground pepper
- 1 tsp chilli flakes

METHOD

1. Put all the ingredients into a food processor and mix until it starts binding together. It will look like dough.
2. Using a tablespoon as your measure, place 1 spoon at a time on a baking sheet lined with baking paper. Press the mixture flat.
3. Bake at 200°C for 10 minutes.
4. If they are still pale on the underside, turn them over and bake for another 3-4 minutes. You want them to be an even, dark colour. Cool on a cooling rack. They should be crispy and light.

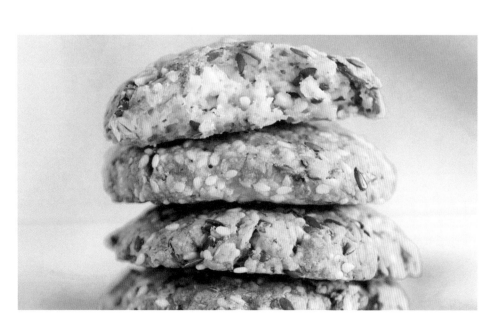

03

COURGETTE BREAD

Makes one loaf

The texture of this bread is fantastic – it does not taste of nut flour or courgettes.

INGREDIENTS

- 5 eggs
- 50ml olive oil
- 4 courgettes (550g), grated
- 20g almond flour (or ground macadamia nuts)
- 30g coconut flour
- 2 tbsp psyllium husk
- 1½ tsp baking powder
- 100g mozzarella, grated
- 85g pumpkin seeds
- 170g mixed seeds of your choice
- 1 tsp salt
- 1 tsp dried mixed herbs

METHOD

1. Preheat the oven to 180°C, and grease a medium-sized loaf pan.
2. Whisk the eggs and olive oil together, add the courgettes and mix well.
3. Add the rest of the ingredients and stir to combine.
4. Pour the mixture into a greased loaf pan.
5. Bake at 180°C in the middle of the oven for 60 minutes. Use a skewer to test that it is cooked through; if it comes out dry, the bread is done.
6. Turn the oven off and allow the bread to cool in the oven for 10-15 minutes to dry.
7. Cool before slicing.

This is a moist bread, so leave in the oven a little longer than you otherwise might. It stores best in a brown paper bag on your worktop.

TIP

For toasted sandwiches, place a filling of your choice between two slices and fry in butter in the pan. Or use a flat sandwich press.

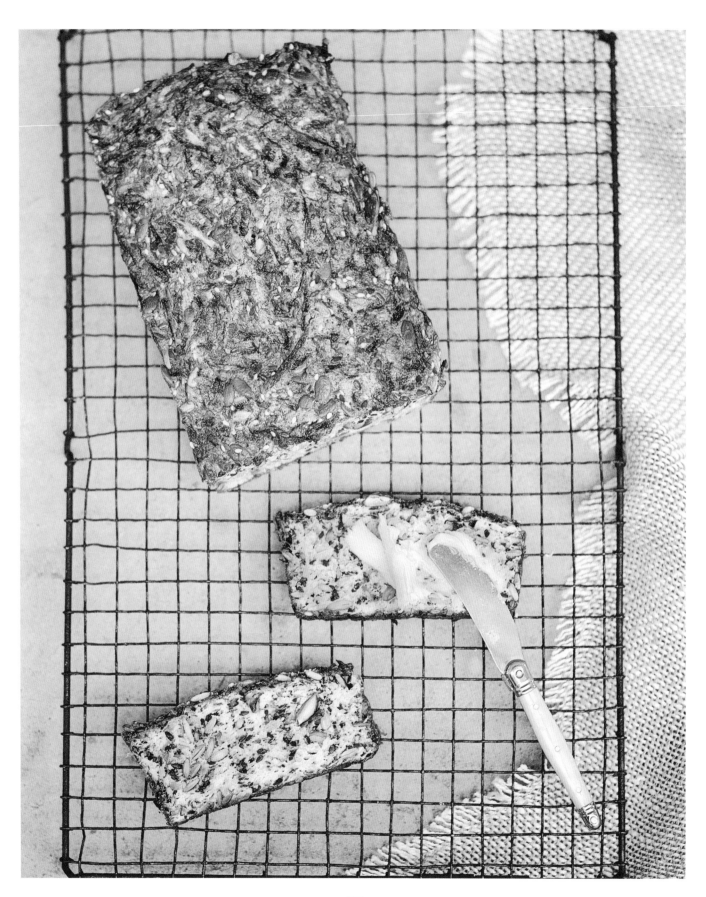

Desserts **01**

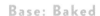

CHOCOLATE CHEESECAKE

Makes 10-12 slices

There are two options for the base: one is baked, the other is refrigerated. Use a springform baking tin so that it is easy to remove when you are ready to serve it.

Base: Baked

INGREDIENTS

- 90g butter, melted
- 80g desiccated coconut
- 75g almond flour
- Pinch of salt

METHOD

1. Mix all ingredients together and press down into a greased springform tin.
2. Bake at 180°C for 10-15 minutes. Remove from oven and cool.

Base: Refrigerated

INGREDIENTS

- 60g desiccated coconut
- 85g pumpkin seeds
- 4 tbsp cocoa powder
- 30g xylitol
- 60g butter

METHOD

1. In a food processor, mix the coconut and pumpkin seeds until fine.
2. Add the cocoa powder and xylitol and pulse to combine.
3. Add the butter, and blend until combined.
4. The mixture will start forming balls in your food processor.
5. Put the mixture into your baking tin, and press it down evenly with the back of a spoon.
6. Let it set in the refrigerator while you make the filling.

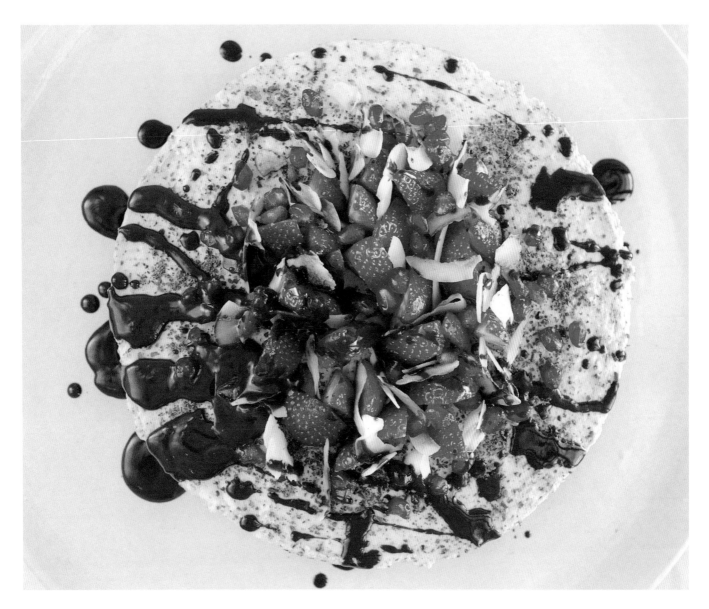

Chocolate filling

INGREDIENTS

- 500g smooth cream cheese
- 1 tsp vanilla extract
- 35g xylitol
- 3 eggs, separated
- 1 tbsp gelatine, powdered
- 50ml cold water
- 100g chocolate, grated
- 250ml cream, whipped

METHOD

1. Beat cream cheese, vanilla and xylitol together.
2. Add egg yolks and beat well.
3. Dissolve the gelatine in water over heat and stir into mixture. Add two-thirds of the chocolate.
4. Whisk the egg whites until meringue-like and fold in; then fold in cream. Spoon into tin.
5. If you didn't add all the chocolate, melt the remaining chocolate and drizzle over the top of cake. Swirl with a knife to give a marbled effect.
6. Refrigerate until set.

02

COURGETTE BROWNIES

Makes 12-16 squares

This recipe may get little Timmy eating courgette for the first time. It keeps very well in the fridge. As it is very rich, you will not need a very big portion.

INGREDIENTS

- 200g courgette, finely grated
- 90g butter, melted
- 2 tbsp coconut oil
- 1 large egg
- 40g xylitol or erythritol
- 65g macadamia nut flour (almond flour also works well)
- 30g cocoa powder
- 1 tsp baking powder
- 50g nuts, chopped – use your favourite variety
- 50g dark chocolate, chopped

METHOD

1. Preheat the oven to 180°C.
2. Mix all the wet ingredients with the xylitol, and then stir in the dry ingredients, including the nuts and half the chocolate.
3. Your batter should be thick but not dry (if the courgette is dry, you may need to add a spoon of water to the batter).
4. Put your mix into a greased brownie tin.
5. Sprinkle the other half of the chocolate on top.
6. Bake for 30 minutes. It should be very moist in the centre.
7. Once cool, score with a knife, and then chill to set before you take the squares out of the pan.
8. This is very decadent served with thick double cream or whipped cream.

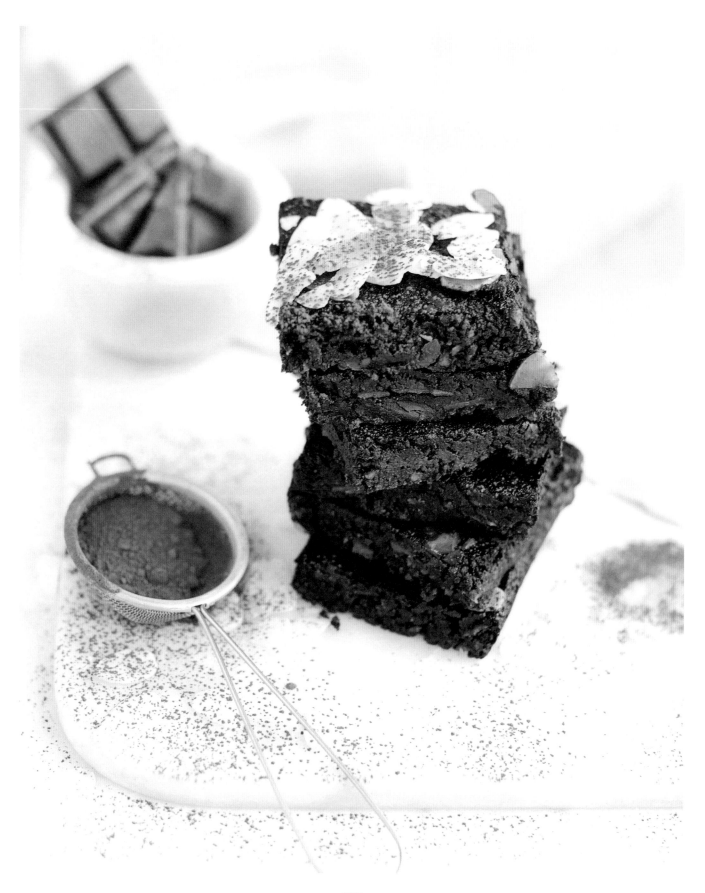

03

CHOCOLATE POTS

Makes 6-8 portions

This is a decadent dairy-free, guilt-free chocolate dessert. The recipe makes 6 generous portions, but because it is so rich you can make smaller portions which will serve 8. This is not a sweet dessert; to sweeten I would recommend adding a couple of tablespoons of xylitol to the mixture, adding the sweetener slowly and according to your taste.

INGREDIENTS

- 100g dark chocolate
- 3 tbsp coconut oil
- 45g butter
- 1 tsp vanilla extract
- 300ml coconut milk
- 2 large eggs

METHOD

1. In a double boiler, melt the chocolate, coconut oil and butter.
2. Remove from the heat and add vanilla extract and coconut milk.
3. Add eggs, one at a time and whisk.
4. Pour the mixture into ramekins.
5. Place them in a roasting pan and pour boiling water to half the depth, cover with aluminium foil and bake at 150°C for 30 minutes.
6. Remove from the oven, cool and then chill in the fridge before serving.
7. Delicious as is, or top with whipped fresh cream and some berries.

TIP

If you don't have a double boiler, use a glass bowl over a pot of hot water.

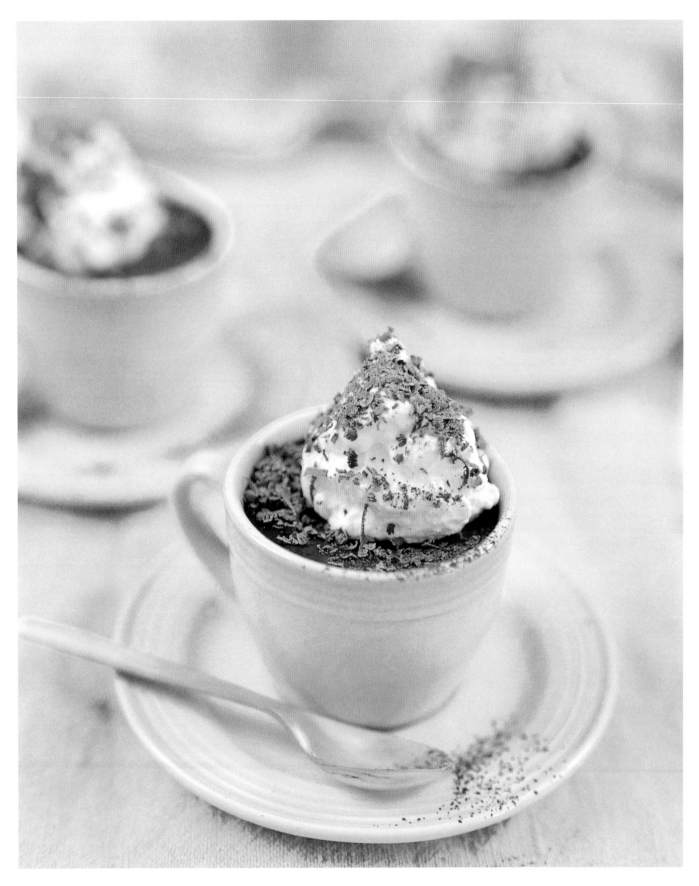

04

CREAMY ICE CREAM

Serves 6

Most people love ice-cream and converting to a low-carb lifestyle doesn't mean you'll have to miss out on your favourite treat. You won't even know that you are eating a low-carb alternative. Once you have the basics right, add your favourite flavours and create toppings.

INGREDIENTS

- 500ml full fat milk (for dairy-free switch for almond milk or coconut milk)
- 250ml double cream (for dairy-free use coconut cream)
- 1 tsp vanilla extract (or a pinch of vanilla powder if preferred)
- 4 egg yolks
- 65g xylitol

METHOD

1. Pour the milk, cream and vanilla into a saucepan, heating slowly and stirring continuously until the milk and cream begin to steam. Reduce the heat to the lowest temperature.
2. Whisk egg yolks together in a glass bowl until smooth. Add the xylitol and whisk until pale yellow and fluffy.
3. Remove the milk from the heat, and slowly pour the steaming milk into the egg mixture, whisking continuously so as not to 'scramble' the eggs. Return the saucepan to the stove and maintain at low heat.
4. Pour the custard mixture into the saucepan from the glass bowl. Continue to heat, stirring continuously until you can coat the back of a wooden spoon with the custard, but do not boil.
5. Remove the custard from the stove; pour into a steel bowl and allow to cool to room temperature, stirring every 10 minutes. Once the custard is cooled, refrigerate overnight (or for at least 6 hours). Never put the hot mixture straight into the fridge.
6. Remove chilled custard mixture from the fridge and place into an ice cream maker. Scoop the ice cream into a freezer-proof container with a lid and freeze for 90 minutes to 2 hours.

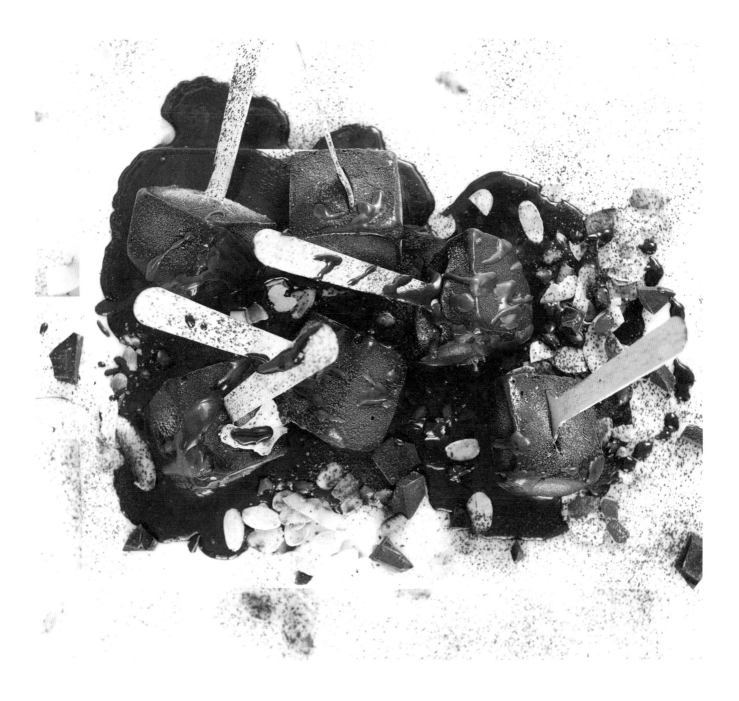

VARIATIONS:

Chocolate – Add 120g sieved cocoa powder and 200g roughly chopped dark chocolate to the steaming milk and stir until blended. Pass through a sieve if necessary. Then add chocolate milk to the egg mixture and return to the heat. You can adjust cocoa and chocolate to your preferred taste.

With caramel sauce – Melt 30g butter on low heat in a pan till light brown. Add 2 tbsp cream, 1 tsp xylitol and a pinch of salt and continue to stir on low heat till sauce has thickened to a caramel (about 1-2 minutes).

Desserts **05**

VANILLA PANNA COTTA WITH BERRY JELLY

Serves 6

Visually, this is a stunning dessert. Both components are delicious and you could make just the panna cotta, or the jelly on its own.

Vanilla panna cotta

INGREDIENTS

- 250ml full-fat Greek yoghurt
- 250ml cream
- 50g xylitol
- 1 tsp vanilla extract
- Pinch of salt
- 200ml full fat milk
- 4 tsp powdered gelatine

METHOD

1. Combine yoghurt, cream, xylitol, vanilla and salt. Stir until combined well.
2. Heat milk until warm (not boiling). Add gelatine. Combine well.
3. Add to cream and yoghurt mixture. Combine well.
4. Strain through fine sieve into pouring jug.
5. Divide equally into 6 beautiful glasses. Chill in freezer until set. Then add berry jelly on top.

Berry jelly

INGREDIENTS

- 400g mixed fresh berries
- 35g xylitol
- 100ml water
- ½ tsp freshly cracked black pepper
- 1 tbsp powdered gelatine

METHOD

1. Combine all ingredients, except gelatine, in a small saucepan.
2. Crush berries with fork. Bring to the boil and boil for 5 minutes.
3. Set aside to cool to just warm. Sprinkle gelatine powder onto berry mixture and stir well.
4. Strain through sieve into pouring jug and pour onto set panna cotta. Chill until the jelly is set.

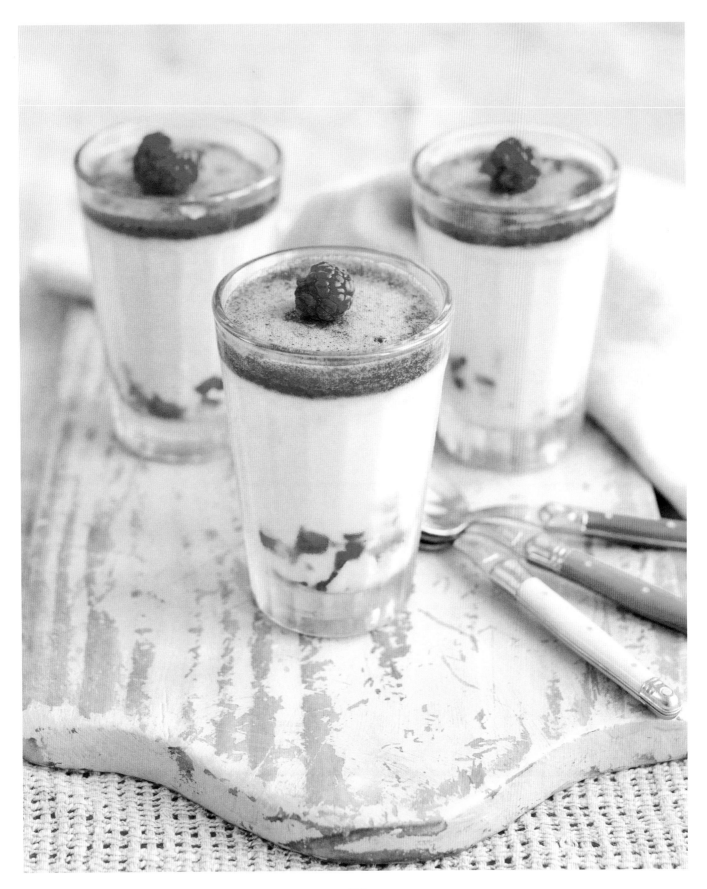

06

MILKSHAKES

Serves 6

A healthy alternative to the usual milkshake, this is a delicious yet sugar-free version of a chocolate milkshake, or the more unusual salted butter milkshake. This may sound odd, but it's delicious. My boys love to meddle in the kitchen and it is encouraged in our house. They developed this shake all on their own and absolutely love it! So, this one's theirs to claim.

Chocolate milkshake

INGREDIENTS

- 360ml ice
- 250ml coconut cream
- 2 tbsp raw cocoa powder
- 2 tbsp xylitol
- 1 tsp vanilla extract

METHOD

1. Place all ingredients into a blender and blitz until smooth and creamy.
2. Pour into glasses.

Salted butter milkshake

INGREDIENTS

- 50g salted butter
- 2 tbsp xylitol
- 1 tsp vanilla extract
- 360ml ice
- 250ml full fat milk (or coconut milk)

For best results use a high-powered blender – one that can crush ice well.

METHOD

1. Melt butter and xylitol in a saucepan.
2. Add vanilla extract and stir well.
3. Place in the blender, add the ice and milk.
4. Blend until ice is crushed, pour into a glass.

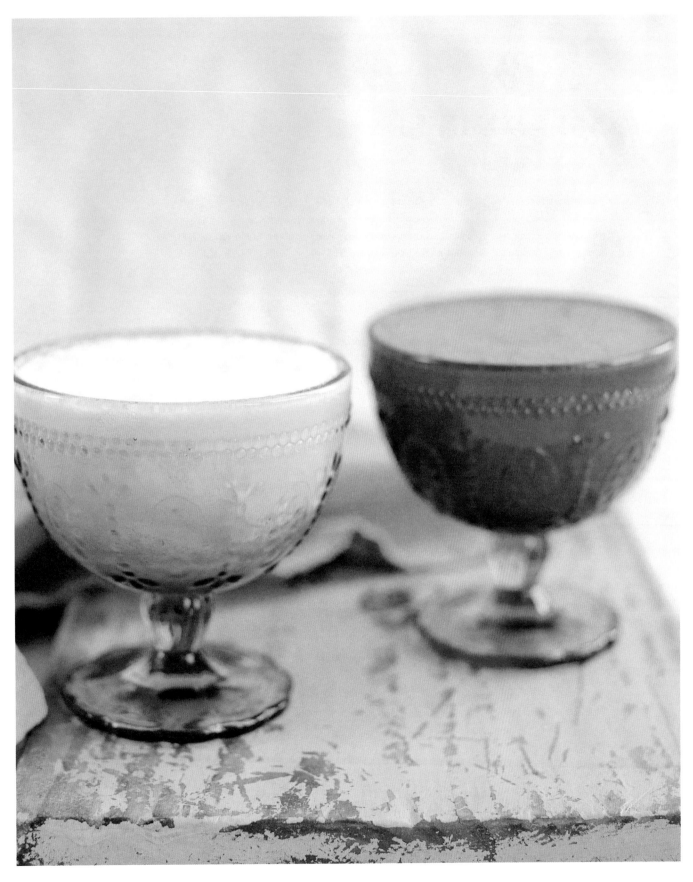

07

BAKED VANILLA CUSTARD

Serves 6

This is a basic recipe that can be altered to suite your needs. For serving at a dinner party, top with toasted almonds or toasted coconut flakes.

INGREDIENTS

- 500ml cream
- 40g xylitol
- 1 tsp vanilla extract
- 5 egg yolks

METHOD

1. Preheat your oven to 160°C and prepare a bain-marie (or use a roasting pan with aluminium foil over the top). You will need 6 ramekins.
2. Heat the cream, xylitol and vanilla until very hot, but not yet boiling.
3. In a separate bowl, beat the egg yolks. Slowly pour the hot liquid over the yolks, whisking constantly. Divide the mixture between the 6 ramekins.
4. Place into a roasting pan and pour boiling water into half the depth of the dish. Bake covered for an hour.

VARIATIONS

- **Coffee-flavoured** – leave out the vanilla and 25ml of cream; replace these with 25ml of espresso (either made with espresso powder or a coffee machine).
- **Chocolate** – along with the vanilla, add 1 tbsp of cocoa powder to the cream mixture. For more decadence, add 50g melted chocolate instead of cocoa powder.

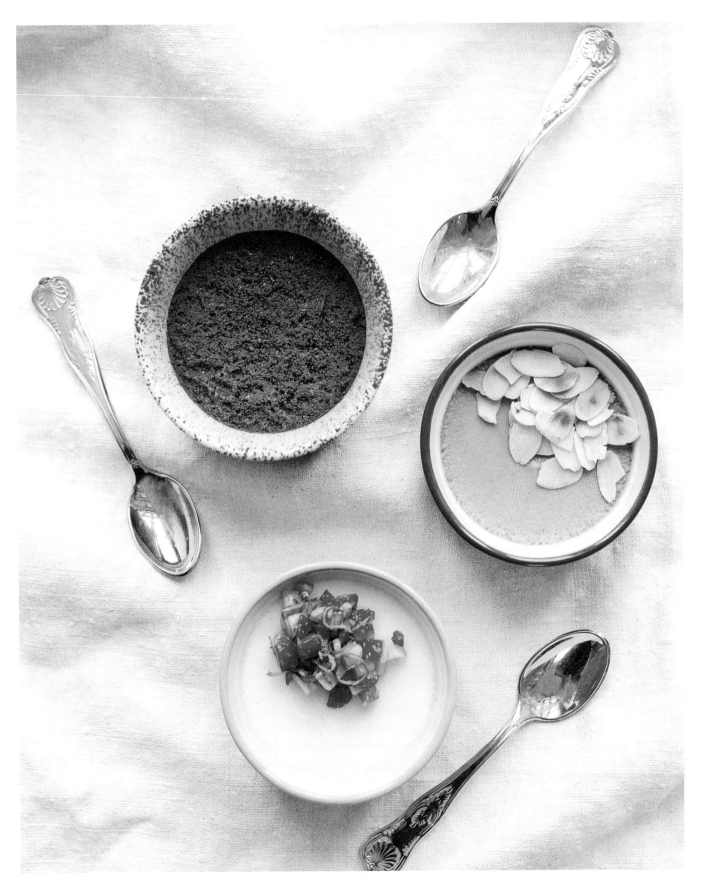

Desserts **08**

CHOCOLATE SAUCE

Serves 4-6

Hands up, who doesn't love chocolate sauce? This one is guilt-free and has a buttery undertone that is simply out of this world.

INGREDIENTS

- 30g butter
- 2 tbsp xylitol
- 1 tsp vanilla extract
- 15g cocoa
- 45g 100% cacao chocolate (substitute with any dark chocolate)

METHOD

1. Melt the butter and xylitol together in a saucepan.
2. Whisk and allow to heat until butter and xylitol appear light yellow. Add vanilla extract and stir.
3. Add the cocoa and chocolate and reduce the heat to lowest temperature, while slowly stirring until melted. To prevent the chocolate from burning, stir slowly.

VARIATIONS

For a chocolate shake
Pour the chocolate sauce into a cup of full fat milk or coconut milk and blend.

For hot chocolate
Warm a cup of milk on the stove until just steaming. Add the chocolate sauce into the milk and stir until mixed.

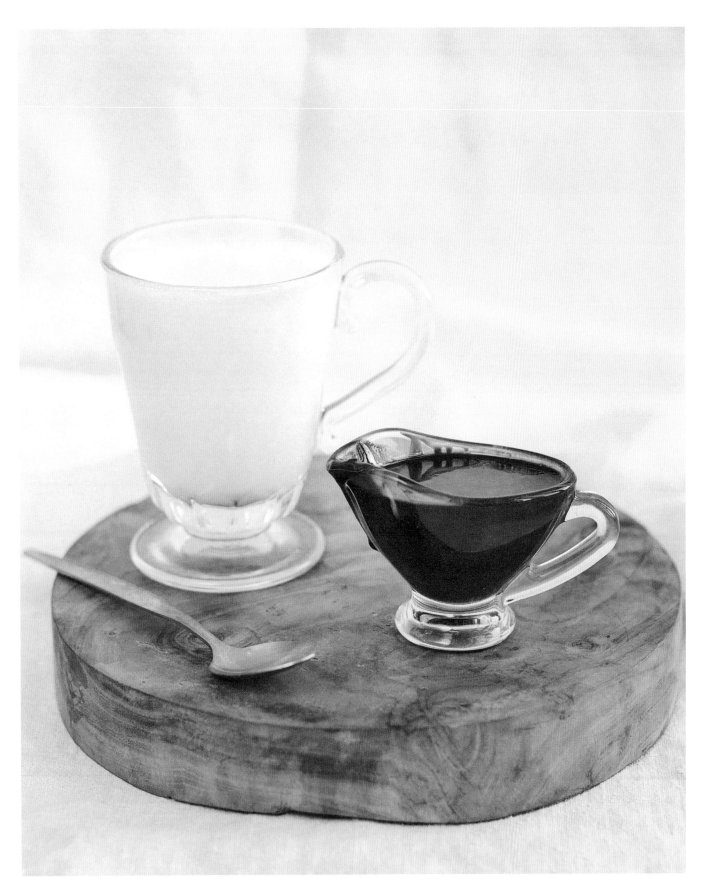

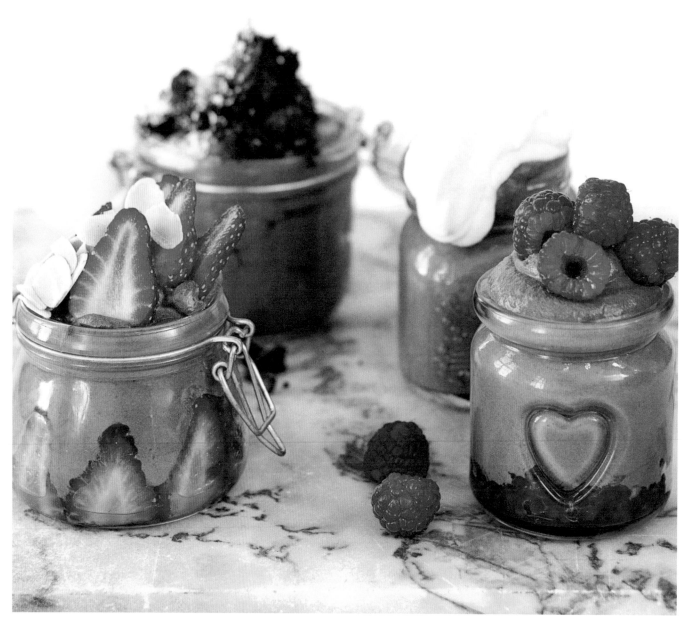

09

LIGHT AND FLUFFY CHOCOLATE MOUSSE

Serves 6-8

There are many mousse recipes about, but this one is so light you will feel as though you are floating away.

INGREDIENTS

- 400ml coconut cream
- 50g cocoa powder
- 50g xylitol
- 2 tsp vanilla extract
- 50g dark chocolate
- 30g butter
- 5 egg whites

METHOD

1. Whisk together coconut cream, cocoa powder, xylitol and vanilla extract.
2. On the stove top, melt the butter and dark chocolate together.
3. Pour the chocolate into the cream mixture and stir well.
4. In a separate bowl, whisk together the egg whites until stiff peaks form.
5. Fold the egg whites into the chocolate mixture a spoonful at a time to keep the mixture light and fluffy.
6. Spoon the mousse into serving glasses or keep in a large bowl and set in the fridge for 20 minutes.
7. Serve chilled.

SERVING SUGGESTIONS:

- Serve with berries, whipped coconut cream or chocolate sauce.
- Crumble some brownies over the mousse.
- Top with berry jelly.

MEDICAL DISCLAIMER

The information and material provided in this document is representative of the opinions and views of Sally-Ann Creed. This body of work is meant for educational and informational purposes only, and is not a substitute for medical advice. It is also not meant to prevent, diagnose, treat or cure any disease condition, nor is any part of the work prescriptive. The content is meant for the sole purpose of furthering knowledge in the field of the low-carbohydrate lifestyle, and should not be construed as medical or dietary advice. The information provided in this work is to be used at the individual's own discretion. Sally-Ann Creed is in no way providing instruction, prescription or professional medical advice and cannot be responsible or held liable for the decisions and actions which may be undertaken as a result of reading her content. Accordingly, the reader agrees that Sally-Ann Creed shall not be liable in any manner for any damage, loss or liability that results from their use of the content of this work or by any third party who obtains the content from the reader. Further, as a reader of this work, the reader agrees to indemnify and hold Sally-Ann Creed harmless from and against any and all claims, losses, liabilities and damages that may arise out of their use of the content of this work. Should the reader need professional medical assistance, a qualified physician or licensed healthcare practitioner should always be immediately consulted. By reading this work, the reader signifies their full acceptance of the above-mentioned terms. Sally-Ann strongly advises that all illnesses are always treated by a qualified medical practitioner and that, before starting any new dietary regimen whatsoever, your medical practitioner is consulted and informed of your decision.

ACKNOWLEDGEMENTS

I am eternally grateful to an amazing man, Dr Robbie Simons in Perth, Australia, who taught me how to regain my health within a few short months. I would probably not be here if he had not intervened at a crucial stage in my life when I was at death's door (my story is related in my seminal work, *Let Food Be Your Medicine*). Wracked with pain, on masses of medication, and with more than one chronic disease, I was treated by Robbie who guided me through the maze of health information and misinformation over twenty years ago. I have never looked back; I have a level of health and energy I never had as a younger person. Robbie was and always will be, my first 'health hero'.

Other heroes along the way for me have been Dr Robert Buist, my mentor and teacher in Syndey, Australia, for his generous friendship and profound work. Dr Jeffrey Bland's work inspired and revolutionised my thinking in the early days, and the works of Dr Barry Sears, Dr Jenny Brand-Miller, Dr Gerald Reaven, Dr Joseph Pizzorno, Dr Matthias Rath and the father of modern medicine, Dr Linus Pauling, all had a profound influence on my early education in the area of health. They have shaped how I understand the concepts and science of health and disease and truly how I live my life. There are hundreds of others who have shaped my education – to each I owe a debt of gratitude as they are the giants on whose shoulders I have stood and still stand today.

In particular I would also like to recognise the work and science of the newly emerging giants in the LCHF world from whom I enjoy learning today. Dr Robert Lustig, Dr Andreas Eenfeldt, Gary Taubes, Dr Jason Fung, Chef Pete Evans, Robb Wolf, Dr Chris Kresser and Nora Gedgaudes – and so many others not mentioned here. To you all – Salut.

A very special thank you goes to Claire Gunn (www.clairegunn.com) for her absolutely beautiful photography, gentle manner, fun in the kitchen while we shot the pictures and for the way she blended into the team as we put the book together. Claire is well known in South Africa as one of the top food photographers, and it's been my honour and privilege to have her shoot this work. Thank you so much Claire, you are a gem.

My profound gratitude also goes to Andrew Burke of Pure Creative (purecreative.co.za, +27 (0) 21 424 6918) for the design and layout of the original version of *The Low-Carb Healthy Fat Bible* (called *The Low-Carb Creed* in South Africa) – for his and his team's dedication to the project, and for going that extra mile. I have seldom seen anyone with so much passion for what he does and clearly loves doing. There was so much thought and love put into this book – my sincere thanks to Andrew and all at Pure Creative for their beautiful and unique work.

To the two delightful contributing authors, Merle Westcott and Janita Bold, I would like to say thank you so much for your amazing recipes and the fun we had putting them together. Merle began as a high school teacher and hasn't lost her passion to teach – she is passionate about this lifestyle and helps to coach others into a healthy LCHF way of life. Janita, owner of a gorgeous wholefood restaurant and mum to three busy boys, began her journey as a diabetic, but due to losing a lot of weight and going LCHF, she is now no longer diabetic. Both Merle and Janita trained under me as LCHF Coaches, and are part of a coaching group I pioneered and established in 2014 – the first LCHF Coaches in the world to my knowledge. Today both Merle and Janita are successful LCHF Coaches and have their health and their figures back! They are inspiring in every sense of the word, and I would like to thank them both for their enthusiasm, sense of fun and lovely recipes. Cheers to you both.

INDEX

BIBLIOGRAPHY

- Abrhams, H.L. "The Relevance of Paleolithic Diet in Determining Contemporary Nutritional Needs." *Evolution Diet*. <www.evolutiondiet.org/Abrams1979PaleolithicNutrition.pdf>
- Adams, A. "What is Potassium Metabisulphite?" *Livestrong*. <www.livestrong.com/article/470024-what-is-potassium-metabisulphite>
- Anton, S.D. *et al*, 2008. "Effects of Chromium Picolinate on Food Intake and Safety." *Diabetes Technology & Therapeutics*. 10(5): 405-412.
- Attia, P., M.D. "Is Ketosis Dangerous?" *The Eating Academy*. <eatingacademy.com/nutrition/is-ketosis-dangerous>.
- Banting, W. 1865. *Letter of Corpulence*. 3rd edition. A Roman & Col: San Francisco.
- Bazinet, R.P. Chu, MWA. 2013. "Omega-6 Polyunsaturated Fatty Acids: Is a Broad Cholesterol-Lowering Health Claim Appropriate?" *Canadian Medical Association Journal*.
- Bowden, J. and Stephen, S. 2012. *The Great Cholesterol Myth: Why Lowering Your Cholesterol Won't Prevent Heart Disease and the Statin-Free Plan that Will*. Fair Winds Press: Beverly, MA.
- Dr Briffa, J. "BMJ Articles Exposes How we've Been Misled Over the 'Benefits' of Statins." *BMJ*. <www.drbriffa.com/2013/11/01/bmj-articles-exposes-the-ways-we-have-been-misled-over-the-benefits-of-statins>
- Browning, J.D. *et al*. "Short-Term Weight Loss and Hepatic Triglyceride Reduction: Evidence of a Metabolic Advantage With Dietary Carbohydrate Restriction." *AmJ Clinical Nutrition*. 93(5):1048-52.
- Bruso, J. "Side Effects of Sodium Cyclamate?" *Livestrong*. <www.livestrong.com/article/332113-side-effects-of-sodium-cyclamate>
- Caldwell, J.G. "Harmful Food Additives." *Foundation Website*. <www.foundationwebsite.org/Miscellany35.pdf>.
- Carillo, A.E. *et al*. 2003. "Impact of Vitamin D Supplementation During a Resistance Training Intervention on Body Composition, Muscle Function, and Glucose Tolerance in Overweight and Obese Adults." *Clin Nutr*. 32(3):375-81.
- Colpo, A. "How I Went From Vegan to Meat Eater and Felt Much Better." *Never Mind the Bollocks, Here's the Science*. <anthonycolpo.com/how-i-went-from-vegan-to-meat-eater-and-felt-much-better>
- Connor, W.E. 2000. "Importance of N-3 Fatty Acids in Health and Disease." *American Journal of Clinical Nutrition*. 71 (suppl):171S-75S.
- Cordain, L. "Beans and Legumes: Are they Paleo?" *The Paleo Diet*. <thepaleodiet.com/beans-and-legumes-are-they-paleo>
- Cromwell, W.C. *et al* .2007. "Clinical Implications of Discordance Between LDL Cholesterol and LDL Particle Number." *J Clin Lipidology*. 1(6):583-592.
- Crowe F.L., *et al*. 2009. "The Association Between Diet and Serum Concentrations of IGF-I, IGFBP-1, IGFBP-2, and IGFBP-3 in the European Prospective Investigation into Cancer and Nutrition." *Cancer Epidemiol Biomarkers Prev*. 18(5):1333-40.
- "CSPI Downgrades Splenda From 'Safe' to 'Caution'". *The Center for Science in the Public Interest*. <www.cspinet.org/new/201306121.html>
- Diamond, J. 2006. *Collapse: How Societies Choose to Succeed or Fail*. Penguin Books: New York.
- Cordain, L. 2012. *The Paleo Answer*. John Wiley & Sons, Hoboken, New Jersey.
- "Daily Protein Requirement." *Ketogenic Diet Resource*. <www.ketogenic-diet-resource.com/daily-protein-requirement.html>
- Daniels, C. "Side Effects of Sodium Cyclamate." *SF Gate*. <healthyeating.sfgate.com/side-effects-sodium-cyclamate-1903.html>
- Daniel, K. 2005. *The Whole Soy Story: The Dark Side of*

America's Favourite Health Food. New Trends Publishing: Washington DC.

- Davidson J.R., *et al.* 1991. "How Sleep Affects Fat-Regulating Hormones: Growth Hormone and Cortisol Secretion in Relation to Sleep and Wakefulness." *J Psychiatry. Neurosci.* 16(2): 96-102.

- Davis, W. 2013. *Wheat Belly.* Rodale: USA.

- Dukan, P. 2010. *The Dukan Diet.* Hodder & Stoughton: London.

- "E Number Index." *The UK Food Guide.* www.ukfoodguide. net/enumeric.htm

- Fallon, S. and Enig, M.G. "The Great Con-ola." *The Weston A Price Foundation.* <www.westonaprice.org/know-your-fats/the-great-con-ola >

- Fallon, S. and Enig, M.G. "The Skinny on Fats." *Weston A Price Foundation.* <www.westonaprice.org>

- "Food E Numbers". *La Leva di Archimede.* <www.laleva.cc/food/xylitol.html >

- Gaziano, J.M., M.D., M.P.H., *et al.* 1997. "Fasting Triglycerides, High-Density Lipoprotein, and Risk of Myocardial Infarction". *Circulation.* American Heart Association. 96:2520-2525.

- Gillespie, D. "How Margarine Breaks your Bones." *David Gillespie.* <davidgillespie.org/how-margarine-breaks-your-bones>

- Glenning, C. "Fat Trims your Waistline." *Corren.* <www.corren.se/ostergotland/fett-ger-fett-smal-midja-6553250-artikel.aspx>

- Green, N. "Moderation is Health! Oleic Sunflower Oil Adverse Effects." *Oilypedia.* <oilypedia.com/moderation-is-health-high-oleic-sunflower-oil-adverse-effects>

- Greer S.M., *et al.* 2013. "The Impact of Sleep Deprivation on Food Desire in the Human Brain." *Nat Commun.* 4(2259).

- Griggs, J. "Are Alzheimer's and Diabetes the Same Disease?" *New Scientist.* <www.newscientist.com/article/mg22029453-400-are-alzheimers-and-diabetes-the-same-disease>

- Hanlon, E.C. PhD., *et al.* "Sleep Restriction Enhances the Daily Rhythm of Circulating Levels of Endocannabinoid 2-Arachidonoylglycerol." *Sleep.* <www.journalsleep.org/ViewAbstract.aspx?pid=30492>

- Heine, R.J., *et al.* "Management of Hyperglycemia in Type 2 Diabetes." *BMJ.* 2006.333:1200. <www.bmj.com/content/333/7580/1200?page=1&tab=responses#alternate>

- Hendrickson, K. "Foul Body Odor from Going on the Atkins Diet?" *Livestrong.* <www.livestrong.com/article/360408-foul-body-odor-from-going-on-the-atkins-diet>

- Hope, J. "Diabetes Danger in Just one Sugary Drink a Day: Chance of Developing Type 2 Increases By A Fifth." *The Daily Mail.* <www.dailymail.co.uk/health/article-2314353/Diabetes-danger-just-ONE-sugary-drink-day-Chance-developing-Type-2-increases-fifth.html>

- Hope, J. "Is a High-Fat Diet Good for the Heart? Doctors say Cars are More Damaging to the Arteries than Butter or Cream." *The Daily Mail.* <www.dailymail.co.uk/health/article-2472672/Is-high-fat-diet-GOOD-heart-Doctors-say-carbs-damaging-arteries.html>

- Hu, J.S. "Aspartame – Other Sweetnesrs." *Sweet Poison.* <www.sweetpoison.com/aspartame-sweeteners.html>

- "Interview with an Ex-Vegan: Denise Minger." *Let Them Eat Meat.* <letthemeatmeat.com/post/1438446275/interview-with-an-ex-vegan-denise-minger>

- Jacobs, J. "What Foods Contain Benzoic Acid?" *Livestrong.* <www.livestrong.com/article/517967-what-foods-contain-benzoic-acid>

- Jaret, P. "Almost Everything you Know About Saturated Fat is Wrong." *More.* <www.more.com/health/healthy-eating/saturated-fat-good>

- Keith, L. 2009. *The Vegetarian Myth.* Flashpoint Press.

- "Ketoacidosis versus Ketosis." *Ketogenic Diet Resource.* <www.ketogenic-diet-resource.com/ketoacidosis.html>

- Kendrick, M. 2007. *The Great Cholesterol Con.* John Blake Publishing, London.

- Kerr, G. "What Are the Dangers of Potassium Sorbate?" *Jillian Michaels.* <livewell.jillianmichaels.com/dangers-potassium-sorbate-5048.html>

- Knutson, K. *et al.* 2005. "Physiology and Pathophysiology of Sleep Apnea Sleep Loss: A Novel Risk Factor for Insulin Resistance and Type 2 Diabetes." *J Appl Physiol.* 99:2008-19.

- Kramer, J. "The Health Effects of BHA and BHT on your Body." *Woodbury Patch.* <patch.com/minnesota/woodbury/bp--the-health-effects-of-bha-and-bht-on-your-body>

- Kresser, C. "Are you Lower-Carb Than you Think?" *Chris Kresser.* <chriskresser.com/are-you-lower-carb-than-you-think>

- Kresser, C. "Why you Should Think Twice About Vegetarian or Vegan Diets." *Chris Kresser*. <chriskresser.com/why-you-should-think-twice-about-vegetarian-and-vegan-diets>
- "Krill." *National Geographic*. <animals.nationalgeographic.com/animals/invertebrates/krill.html>
- Larosa J.C., *et al*. 1980. "With FFAs Being Liberated From Dietary Fat And Body Fat Into the Blood Effects of High-Protein, Low-Carbohydrate Dieting on Plasma Lipoproteins and Body Weight." *J Am Diet Assoc*. 77: 264-270.
- Leproult R. *et al*. 1997. Sleep Loss Results in an Elevation of Cortisol Levels the Next Evening. *Sleep*. 20(10):865-70.
- Longo, N. "Cardiologist Speaks Out on the Myth of Bad Saturated Fat, Stating Carbs are More Damaging Than Butter." *Coconut Oil*. <coconutoil.com/cardiologist-speaks-out-on-the-myth-of-bad-saturated-fat-stating-carbs-are-more-damaging-than-butter>
- "Low-Carb Side Effects & How to Cure Them." *DietDoctor*. <www.dietdoctor.com/low-carb/side-effects>
- Lustig, R. 2013. *Fat Chance*. Fourth Estate, London.
- Lyden, E. "Artificial Sweeteners: Why You Should Completely Avoid them to Stay Healthy." Policy Mic. <www.mic.com/articles/16014/artificial-sweeteners-why-you-should-completely-avoid-them-to-stay-healthy#.9eP3u64pT>
- Mamur, S. *et al*. "Does Potassium Sorbate Induce Genotoxic or Mutagenic Effects in Lymphocytes?" *Toxicology in Vitro*. 24(3). 790-794. <www.sciencedirect.com/science/article/pii/S0887233309003853>
- McClees, H. "Preserving our Food Without Additives: 5 Natural Ingredients that Work Better." *One Green Planet*. <www.onegreenplanet.org/vegan-food/preserving-food-with-natural-ingredients>
- McDonald, L. 1998. The Ketogenic Diet: A Complete Guide for the Dieter and Practitioner. Self-published.
- Mercola, J. "Aspartame's Hidden Dangers." *Mercola*. www.mercola.com/article/aspartame/hidden_dangers.htm
- Mercola, J. "The Potential Dangers of Sucralose." *Mercola*. <www.articles.mercola.com/sites/articles/archive/2000/12/03/sucralose-dangers.aspx>
- Minger, D. 2013. *Death by Food Pyramid*. Malibu, CA. Primal Blueprint Publishing.
- Minger, D. "The China Study Myth." *The Weston A Price Foundation*. <www.westonaprice.org/health-topics/abcs-of-nutrition/the-china-study-myth>
- Moore, J. and Westman, E. 2013. *Cholesterol Clarity*. Victory Belt Publishing Inc: USA.
- "Nutrition Tips to Help you Get Ahead!" *Nature Optimized*. <www.natureoptimized.com/blogs/news/14530409-nutrition-tips-to-help-you-get-ahead >
- Oppenheimer, R.W. 1917. *Diabetic Cookery: Recipes and Menus*. EP Dutton & Company: New York.
- Otvos, J.D., 2002. "Measurement Issues Related to Lipoprotein Heterogeneity." *Am J Cardiol*. 90(suppl): 22i-29i.
- Perlmutter, D. and Loberg, K. 2013. *Grain Brain*. Little, Brown and Company: New York.
- Perlmutter, D. 2015. *Brain Maker*. Yellow Kite: UK.
- "Ratnayake, W.M. *et al*. "Vegetable Oils High in Phytosterols Make Erythrocytes Less Deformable and Shorten the Life Span of Stroke-Prone Spontaneously Hypertensive Rats." *J Nut*. 130(5):1166-78.
- Ravnskov, U. 2009. *Fat and Cholesterol are Good for You*. GB Publishing: Sweden.
- Rheaume-Bleue, K. 2013. *Vitamin K2 and the Calcium Paradox*. Harper Collins.
- Robinson, A.M. 1980. "Physiological Roles of Ketone Bodies as Substrates and Signals in Mammalian Tissues." *DH Williamson Physiological Reviews*. 60(1):143-187.
- Rosenblum, J.L. *et al*. "Calcium and Vitamin D Supplementation is Associated With Decreased Abdominal Visceral Adipose Tissue in Overweight and Obese Adults." *National Center for Biotechnology Information*. <www.ncbi.nlm.nih.gov/pubmed/22170363>
- Rothberg, M.B. "Cardiovascular Perspective: Coronary Artery Diseases as Clogged Pipes." *Circulation*. <www.circoutcomes.ahajournals.org/content/6/1/129>
- Salehpour, A. *et al*. "A 12-Week Double-Blind Randomized Clinical Trial of Vitamin D3 Supplementation on Body Fat Mass in Healthy Overweight and Obese Women." *The Nutrition Journal*. <www.nutritionj.biomedcentral.com/articles/10.1186/1475-2891-11-78>
- Schmid S.M. *et al*. 2008. "A Single Night of Sleep

Deprivation Increases Ghrelin Levels and Feelings of Hunger in Normal-Weight Healthy Men". *J Sleep Res.* 17(3):331-4.

· Schmid, S.M. *et al.* 2009. "Mild Sleep Restriction Acutely Reduces Plasma Glucagon Levels in Healthy Men." *J Clin Endocrinol Metab.* 94(12):5169-73.

· Simpson N.S. *et al.* 2010. "Effects of Sleep Restriction on Adiponectin Levels in Healthy Men And Women". *Physiol Behav.* 101(5):693-8.

· "Select Committee on GRAS Substances (SCOGS) Opinion: Potassium Metabisulfite, Sodium Bisulfite, Sodium Metabisulfite, Sodium Sulfite, Sulfur Dioxide." *FDA.* <www.fda.gov/Food/IngredientsPackagingLabeling/GRAS/SCOGS/ucm261009.htm>

· Sellman, S. "Xylitol: Our Sweet Salvation?" *La Leva di Archimede.* <www.laleva.cc/food/enumbers/E901-970.html>

· Smith, A. *et al.* "Oxidative and Thermal Stabilities of Genetically Modified High Oleic Sunflower Oil." *Research Gate.* <www.researchgate.net/publication/223238589_Oxidative_and_thermal_stabilities_of_genetically_modified_high_oleic_sunflower_oil>

· Smith, S. *et al.* "Oxidative and Thermal Stabilities of Genetically Modified High Oleic Sunflower Oil." *ScienceDirect.* www.sciencedirect.com/science/article/pii/S0308814606005735.

· "Sodium Cyclamate? The Side Effects Could Kill! (Apparently)." *Energy Drinks.* <www.truthaboutenergydrinks.wordpress.com/2011/11/18/sodium-cyclamate-the-side-effects-could-kill-apparently>

· "Some 'Healthy' Vegetable Oils May Actually Increase Risk of Heart Disease." *Science Daily.* <www.sciencedaily.com/releases/2013/11/131111122105.htm>

· Smith, J. 2003. *Seeds of Deception.* Yes! Books: Fairfield, IA.

· Spiegel, K. *et al.* 2004. "Leptin Levels are Dependent on Sleep Duration: Relationships with Sympathovagal Balance, Carbohydrate Regulation, Cortisol, and Thyrotropin." *J Clin Endocrinol Metab.* 89(11):5762-71

· Spiegel, K. *et al.* 2005. "Sleep Loss: A Novel Risk Factor for Insulin Resistance and Type 2 Diabetes." *J Appl Physiol.* 99(5):2008-19.

· "Sweden Touts Low-Carb Diet as Key to Weight Loss." *The Local SE.* <www.thelocal.se/20130923/50384>

· Taubes, G. 2009. *The Diet Delusion.* Knopf of Random House: USA.

· Taubes, G. 2011. *Why We Get Fat and What to do About it.* Knopf of Random House: New York.

· Teicholz, N. 2014. *Big Fat Surprise.* Scribe Publications: Australia.

· Tendler, D. *et al.* "The Effect of a Low Carbohydrate, Ketogenic Diet on NAFLD: A Pilot Study." *Digestive Diseases and Science.* <www.link.springer.com/article/10.1007%2Fs10620-006-9433-5>

· "Two Preservatives to Avoid." *Berkeley Wellness.* <www.berkeleywellness.com/healthy-eating/food-safety/article/two-preservatives-avoid>

· USDA Database <ndb.nal.usda.gov> or Nutridata <www.nutridata.com> (linked to USDA) unless no reference could be found, in which case we have used other reliable sources.

· Watson, A. *Illustrated History of Heart Disease 1825-2015.* Diet Heart Publishing. <dietheartnews.com/2012/08/heart-disease-american-heart-association-diet-heart-hypothesis>

· Weintraub, K. 2014. "We need more sleep". *The Boston Globe.* <www.bostonglobe.com/lifestyle/health-wellness/2014/01/13/sleep-more-important-than-you-might-think/1R6iiCYWbCSKY1K2wmwOVP/story.html>

· Wells, S.D. "Sweetener Warning: Acesulfame Potassium Contains Methylene Chloride, a Known Carcinogen. *Natural News.* <www.naturalnews.com/041510_Acesulfame-K_methylene_chloride_carcinogen.html>

· Yamauchi, T. *et al.* "The Fat-Derived Hormone Adiponectin Reverses Insulin Resistance Associated with Both Lipoatrophy and Obesity." *Nat Med.* 7(8):941-6.

· Yoquinto, L. "The Truth about Food Additive BHA." *Live Science.* <www.livescience.com/36424-food-additive-bha-butylated-hydroxyanisole.html>

YouTube clips

· *Allan Savory: How to Green the World's Deserts and Reverse Climate Change.* www.youtube.com/watch?v=vpTHi7O66pl

· *Alessio Fasano, MD: The Gut is Not Like Las Vegas.* www.youtube.com/watch?v=wha30RSxE6w

- *Alzheimer's / Dementia; Dr. Grant Anderson, Robb Wolf and Dr Peter Attia.* www.youtube.com/watch?v=vxI1NPk1NIg
- *Big Fat Lies,* www.youtube.com/watch?v=v8WA5wcaHp4
- *Carbohydrate and Saturated Fat: Emerging Research and New Schools of Thought.* www.youtube.com/watch?v=4eVZmBMgff0
- *Carbovore to Carnivore: Taming the Carb Craving Monster. Nora Gedgaudas.* www.youtube.com/watch?v=lUen3G4J7U4
- *David Gillespie.* www.youtube.com/watch?v=9CsyX3myOIg
- *David Gillespie: Sweet Poison and Big Fat Lies.* www.youtube.com/watch?v=kVjqfieegB4
- *David Gillespie: Sweet Poison Quit Plan.* www.youtube.com/watch?v=WLIuKT0wBFA
- *Dr Jonny Bowden. "The Great Cholesterol Myth".* www.youtube.com/watch?v=YGOpjPNtjes
- *Dr Mercola Interviews Dr Richard Johnson on Fructose.* www.youtube.com/watch?v=ZjG5t4LN0jA
- *Dr Peter Attia - The Straight Dope on Cholesterol and Diet.* www.youtube.com/watch?v=dAWdHYSrh7M
- *Dr. Richard Bernstein (Part 1) Nutrition & Metabolism Society Meeting.* www.youtube.com/watch?v=9VaNJO7KMgg
- *Enjoy Eating Saturated Fats: They're Good for You. Donald W. Miller, Jr, MD.* www.youtube.com/watch?v=vRe9z32NZHY
- *How Grass-fed Beef will Save the World.* www.youtube.com/watch?v=yxMNHsK-lpI
- *How to Win an Argument with a Vegetarian by Denise Minger.* vimeo.com/27792352
- *How Canola Oil is Made.* www.youtube.com/watch?v=Cfk2IXlZdbI
- *How it's Made: Canola Oil,* www.youtube.com/watch?v=omjWmLG0EAs&feature=youtu.be&t=47s
- *How Sugar is Killing Us... Slowly but Surely with Dr. Aseem Malhotra.* www.youtube.com/watch?v=7dOijIbtGsI
- *Is Potassium Sorbate Bad for You?* nutritionfacts.org/video/is-potassium-sorbate-bad-for-you
- *Joel Salatin — Folks This Ain't Normal!* www.youtube.com/watch?v=IkC3pl5taMs
- *The Oiling of America.* www.youtube.com/watch?v=fvKdYUCUca8
- *Raw Vegan Diet Warning from Denise Minger & RawBrahs.* www.youtube.com/watch?v=Ft_SqZuvhME
- *The Science and Practice of Low-Carb Diets {Duke University Office Hours}.* www.youtube.com/watch?v=toLvGpk3HLE
- *Sugar Dangers - Dr. Richard Johnson Lecture (Part 1 of 3),* www.youtube.com/watch?v=OOJ3SiRj4AQ
- *Colin Campbell v Eric C Westman - Diet Doctors.* www.youtube.com/watch?v=mJYlXmfb08M
- *Uffe Ravnskov: The cholesterol campaign and its misleading dietary advices.* www.youtube.com/watch?v=pMf3aFSdNag
- *The Vegetarian Myth.* www.youtube.com/watch?v=rNON5iNf07o
- *Vitamin D and Prevention of Chronic Diseases.* www.youtube.com/watch?v=Cq1t9WqOD-0
- *William Davis – Wheat: The Unhealthy Whole Grain.* www.youtube.com/watch?v=UbBURnqYVzw
- *Why We Get Fat: Diet Trends and Food Policy.* www.youtube.com/watch?v=UMQKtvj1htU

Reference Websites

- *Alan Watson,* dietheartnews.com
- *Andreas Eenfeldt,* www.dietdoctor.com
- *Chris Kresse,* www.chriskresser.com
- *Denise Minger,* www.rawfoodsos.com
- *Ditch the Carbs,* www.ditchthecarbs.com
- *Fooducate,* www.fooducate.com
- *Jason Fung,* www.intenstivedietarymanagement.com
- *Kris Gunners,* authoritynutrition.com
- *Mark Sisson,* www.marksdailyapple.com
- *Marty Kendall,* www.optimisingnutrition.wordpress.com
- *Nutra Ingredients,* www.nutraingredients.com
- *Peter Attia, The Eating Academy,* www.eatingacademy.com
- *Sarah Ballantyne, The Paleo Mom,* www.thepaleomom.com
- *Statin Nation,* www.statinnation.net
- *Stephen Sinatra,* www.drsinatra.com
- *WebMD.* www.webmd.com
- *Wellness Mama,* wellnessmama.com
- *Weston A Price Foundation,* www.westonaprice.org

CONVERSIONS

IMPERIAL	METRIC	AMERICAN
½ fl oz	15 ml	1 tablespoon
1 fl oz	30 ml	⅛ cup
2 fl oz	60 ml	¼ cup
4 fl oz	120 ml	½ cup
8 fl oz	240 ml	1 cup
16 fl oz	480 ml	1 pint

4oz	100g	
7oz	200g	
10oz	300g	
13oz	400g	
1lb	500g	

In British, Australian and often Canadian recipes an imperial pint is 20 fl oz. American recipes use the American pint measurement, which is 16 fl oz.

NOTES

NOTES

NOTES

NOTES